Babies

ARE NOT

PIZZAS

Babies

ARE NOT

PIZZAS

THEY'RE *BORN*, NOT *DELIVERED!*

REBECCA DEKKER,
PHD, RN

EVIDENCE BASED BIRTH

Cover Photography by The Malicotes
Cover design by Angela Baxter
Book Cover design copyrighted by Evidence Based Birth®
Typeset by Deborah Spencer
Edited by Cristen Pascucci and Rochelle Deans

ISBN-13: 978-1-7325496-6-1

10 9 8 7 6 5 4 3 2 1

Contents

Author's Note

THIS BOOK IS NOT MEANT to advocate for one way of giving birth. The definition of evidence based care includes a) having research-based information to help you make decisions; b) finding a health care provider who can help you interpret that research evidence; and c) considering your own values, goals, and preferences. Since all of us are unique, there is no one right decision for everyone.

We each have our own birth story to tell. Some stories are empowering; others are traumatic; most are unforgettable. Some people feel that the hospital saved their lives. Others view themselves as victims of medical mistakes or unnecessary interventions.

This book contains my story.

Chapter One

NAIVE

I WENT INTO MY FIRST BIRTH with rose-colored glasses. I figured everything would be fine as long as I had a healthy pregnancy—which to me meant exercising and not gaining too much weight.

I had seen a few births back in nursing school, and I didn't want to be one of *those* patients they gossiped about at the nurse's station. So, one of my main goals for this birth was for the nurses to like me—especially because I was giving birth at the hospital affiliated with the university where I was finishing my PhD in Nursing—the only place my student health insurance would permit me to give birth. I planned to listen to my health care providers and do as I was told.

I didn't do too much preparation. I read several popular pregnancy books, which, in retrospect, weren't the best choices. Like the one-day hospital childbirth class my husband Dan and I took, the books seemed to send the message that we should passively accept everything that would be done to us during our hospital stay.

With only random bits of education, I was not prepared for what the system had in store for me. I laughed at birth plans. "How can you possibly 'plan' birth? You're supposed to be *flexible*! You should do what your doctor says—they're the one with the medical degree!"

My only true desire was to have a vaginal birth, and maybe try to avoid pain medication for as long as possible because I am not a fan of needles.

Looking back, I realize I placed total control of my birth into the hands of the professionals who would be taking care of me. What I didn't know then is that if you give up total control of your decisions and don't do any education or planning, you often end up getting the lowest quality of health care, at the highest cost to yourself, your health, and your wallet.

Although I was oblivious about what I was headed toward, my younger sister by two-and-a-half years, Shannon, was really worried for me. Shannon was training to be a doctor in Michigan at the time, and she was witnessing all kinds of concerning situations on the labor and delivery unit. She noticed how many women were receiving totally unnecessary interventions—like medications given to speed up labor even when labor was progressing normally, or episiotomies or Cesareans being done because the physician was tired of waiting for the client to push the baby out. One time a resident told Shannon, "Well, she's 4 centimeters now, so we are going to go break her water."

"Why?" Shannon asked.

Pause. "Because that's what we do."

Feeling a bit like a two-year-old, Shannon again asked, "Why?"

"Because it will make it go faster."

"Why do we need it to go faster?"

The resident grew more annoyed and brushed Shannon off. A few hours later, after finding all the research articles she could on PubMed, Shannon came back to the resident.

"So, I was looking up this issue of rupturing membranes. It looks like it doesn't really make the first stage of labor go faster, and it can increase the risk of infection."[1,2]

As you can probably guess, my sister was not the best-loved student on this rotation. But she did learn a lot about the culture of labor and delivery, and the need for change. Years later, she also told me, "While training in obstetrics, I began to see that we, as doctors, can lie to our patients, and lie to ourselves, if we need to."

Given what she was seeing in the clinical setting, Shannon worried for me, but she didn't tell me horror stories, or preach at me, or tell me what to do. I remember one time, when we were on the phone, she asked some concerned questions about my childbirth preparation, but I brushed her off, saying, "Don't worry about me, I'll be fine!"

I really liked my OB. She was funny, nice, and smart. My husband and I both enjoyed our appointments with her, and she promised that she would be the one present at my birth. I didn't realize at the time how rare my situation was. What my OB offered at the time, and very few OBs practice today, is called continuity of care—when the caregiver at your birth is the person you've been seeing throughout pregnancy. These days, most physicians, out of practical necessity, rotate call, meaning they take turns going to the hospital when someone is in labor. My OB practiced continuity of care with me, and thus she was present at a birth that, in the hands of one of the other OBs in her practice, might have easily become a Cesarean.

I was 39 weeks and 3 days into my pregnancy in the fall of 2008. I had been totally healthy, with the exception of my migraine headaches, which had worsened during pregnancy. Dan and I had finished watching a movie when, just before 11 p.m., my water broke. I felt this little "pop" and a tiny gush of water, like I'd just barely wet my pants.

"I think my water just broke," I exclaimed.

One of the instruction sheets we had been given said to go to the hospital if my water broke, so we started gathering our things. I took a quick shower and ate a big snack, knowing that I wouldn't be allowed to eat or shower once I got to the hospital. I was prepared to obey hospital policy without question—remember, I wanted to be a "good patient." During our quick seven-minute drive to the hospital, my contractions started. They were easy to handle and coming 5 minutes apart.

Dan dropped me off at the hospital entrance and I made my way to triage alone while he parked the car. Triage is sort of a hospital "holding area" for patients coming in for birth—not used in all facilities—where people in labor can be assessed before being admitted. In triage, I was put on a narrow stretcher in a room with another patient, separated only by a curtain. There I was checked in by a nurse, physically examined (including my vagina), asked questions (the other patient could hear my answers), poked for an IV, and hooked up to monitors. During my time in triage, the OB resident took some fluid from my vagina, then hunched over a microscope with a medical student, examining the sample.

"See that fern pattern on the slide? That's amniotic fluid," I remember her telling the excited medical student.

"Wow," the student said breathlessly.

After proving that my water had indeed broken, they signed the paperwork to admit me to the labor and delivery unit.

The triage nurse put me in a wheelchair and wheeled me to L&D. She dropped me off inside the room and said, "You should go to the bathroom now, because you're not allowed to get out of bed from now on."

I remember being struck by that command. It seemed odd, that they didn't plan on letting me use the bathroom while I was in labor, but, desiring to be a compliant patient, I padded my hospital-slippered feet to the bathroom, peed, and returned to the bed. There, I had an IV hooked up to a bag of fluids, a belt fitted tightly around my abdomen to measure my contractions, and another belt placed to measure my baby's heart rate. The belts had these hard, circular shaped discs that pressed firmly and uncomfortably into my very pregnant abdomen.

An hour later, I needed to pee again, and when I pushed the call light button, I was told that I must use a bedpan. Although I'd helped many patients use one in my career, I'd never personally urinated in a bedpan before. I tried, and cannot tell you how difficult it was to urinate lying flat on my back on that hard, plastic pan, while having contractions, with two people watching me! I just could not go. So, the nurse inserted a painful catheter (tube) into my urethra to empty my bladder—instead of letting me walk 10 feet to the bathroom.

Just like that, I had transformed from a healthy pregnant woman to a patient in a hospital gown, lying on my back in a hospital bed. I was offered Pitocin® (artificial oxytocin[3]), a medication used to speed up contractions, but I politely declined. My contractions were already coming 5 minutes apart, so I didn't see the need.

I was beginning to feel a little bit trapped—realizing that I was about to undergo labor without food, drink, movement, or permission to use the bathroom. By now, it was the middle of the night and I was left alone. I knew labor might take a while, so I had told Dan to try to sleep while he could. He slept in an armchair and I endured labor in bed, on my back, in the dark, with a random football game replaying on the TV, and nobody there to support me.

Suddenly, just before sunrise, everything changed. The OB residents, medical student, and attending obstetrician started taking turns rounding on me. I started getting more and more pressure to get Pitocin® and an epidural.

"Your labor's taking an abnormally long time," a resident explained to me around 7 a.m. My water had broken 8 hours earlier. I learned later that it's normal for a first-time mom to have a long early phase of labor, especially if water broke before labor began.[4] But I hadn't gotten past 2 centimeters yet, and they were not happy with my progress.

I hadn't expected to get that kind of pressure. I kept saying, "No, thank you," "No, thank you," "No, thank you," to almost everyone who entered the room. For someone who hadn't had much education about childbirth, I was pretty good at saying "No" to an unnecessary intervention. But, in labor, under pressure, and with no way out except to have the baby, I couldn't say "No" forever.

Around noon, I begrudgingly agreed to the Pitocin®. They started with a low dose, and my labor picked up almost immediately. I had heard that Pitocin®-induced contractions were more painful, so I asked for an epidural. The anesthesiology resident came in to do the procedure. He informed me of the medical benefits and risks of an epidural, and I signed the consent form. However, what happened next was somewhat traumatic. The resident tried once, twice, three times to get the huge needle in my back, but he claimed that because of my scoliosis (mild curve in my spine) and what he described as "tiny bone structure," he couldn't get it in. Those three attempts were excruciatingly painful. Finally, the attending came in to take over and was able to get the epidural placed. Afterward, I shivered uncontrollably, dry heaved, and cried. I couldn't stop crying for a while. I don't know why.

The epidural kicked in. In fact, the nerve block was so strong that I was completely numb from the waist down. I couldn't move my legs at all. Every time I wanted to shift my position, Dan had to move my body around for me. They didn't feel like my own limbs—they felt like elephant legs. It was a weird and uncomfortable sensation. This problem doesn't happen to everyone who gets an epidural, but too strong of a motor block is a potential side effect of epidurals that I happened to experience.[5]

I lay on my back and more time went by, until all of a sudden I felt the urge to push—it felt like I had intense pressure in my bottom. By now, it was 7 p.m. I pushed the button on my call light and the nursing assistant poked her head in the door.

Excitedly, I told her, "I think I'm ready to push!"

She said, "I'm so sorry. Everyone is in report! You'll just have to wait. We'll be back in half an hour or so."

Frightened by the overwhelming pushing feelings, not knowing what to do, I pushed my epidural button repeatedly, delivering doses that numbed all sensations.

About 30 minutes later, the medical student walked in, dressed from head to toe in bodily fluid protection gear, complete with a plastic face shield, like she was about to start welding or something. A half dozen people followed her.

The staff coached me to push; they put my feet in stirrups and I lay on my back, half sitting up. I couldn't feel a single thing in the lower half of my body—the pushy feeling was gone, due to my overzealous attempts to medicate it. The nurse said, "Now hold your breath and push! ONE TWO THREE FOUR FIVE SIX SEVEN EIGHT NINE TEN and again! ONE TWO THREE FOUR FIVE SIX SEVEN EIGHT NINE TEN! And again! ONE TWO THREE FOUR FIVE SIX SEVEN EIGHT NINE TEN!"

This pushing effort went on for an hour, and I made zero progress. I was too numb to push effectively, if at all. But then, after an hour, my epidural started to wear off. I started pushing with a renewed zeal, but after another hour, my baby's head still wasn't coming down. Then my OB did an exam and discovered that the baby's position was not optimal. Later, I found that this was not a surprising finding, given that I'd just spent nearly 24 hours in a back-lying position that didn't allow the baby space to move down and rotate the way she needed to.

Researchers think that laboring upright and moving around uses gravity to help the baby's head descend into the pelvis in the optimal position for birth.[6]

My doctor asked my permission to maneuver the baby's head into a more favorable position, and I consented. Basically, she inserted her entire hand up my vagina and into my dilated cervix, put her hand on the baby's head, and rotated the baby around. Even though I was still partially numb from the epidural, the pain from this procedure was so intense that I leaned over the side of the bed and vomited. However, after she adjusted my baby's position, I finally started making some progress. It was now my third hour of pushing and I was exhausted, but the baby was coming out. At the very end, the OB asked my permission to use a vacuum suction cup device on my baby's head to help pull her out (called a vacuum-assisted delivery), and, again, I consented.

Finally, at 10:50 p.m., my daughter Clara was born, after 24 hours of labor, including more than 3 hours of pushing. Clara was immediately removed from my sight so she could be suctioned, swaddled, measured, and weighed.

As my OB attended to my needs, checking to see if I needed stitches or not (thankfully, I only needed one stitch), I thanked her.

"Thank you," I said. "Thank you so much, for never even mentioning the word C-section after all those hours."

She said, "You're welcome! I knew you didn't want one. And if a woman can't birth a 6 pound, 8 ounce baby vaginally, there's something wrong with this world."

The birth was done, but my baby was not in the room. Although her Apgar scores were normal (Apgar scores are a way of assessing the health of a baby at birth), after they let me take one photo holding her all bundled up, the hospital staff whisked her away to the nursery for "observation."

Now, this did not make sense. I had accepted without question so much of what the hospital told me to do—I'd fasted for 24 hours, used a bedpan, complied with all their requests and recommendations. But I would not—could not—accept separation from my baby, my own baby, who I had been growing inside my body for the last 9 months and was so eager to meet after a full day and night of labor! Still paralyzed from the waist down due to my epidural, I pushed my call light button every 10 or 15 minutes.

"Where is my baby?"

"When will they bring my baby to me?"

"I need to breastfeed!"

One hour went by. Two hours went by. At two hours, when I checked again to see if she was coming to me, I was told over the intercom, "Oh honey, I'm so sorry. We just gave her a bath and her hair's all wet. We have to wait for her hair to dry!"

Finally, at around 1:30 a.m., nearly three hours after she'd been born, she was brought to me for the first breastfeed. She was sleepy (we'd missed the magical "golden hour" when freshly born babies are still wide awake after birth and ready to bond and breastfeed[7]), and she didn't latch well. The night nurse didn't really know how to help me. She just stood by and watched, while I clumsily tried to latch my drowsy baby onto my breast.

It hurt.

I found out later that since my nurse didn't know how to help me, I hadn't properly latched Clara, and as a result, these first attempts to breastfeed left my nipples cracked and damaged, which would haunt us in the days and weeks to come.

The next morning, we were a hot mess. I had started labor Saturday evening, given birth on Sunday evening, and now it was Monday morning. Dan and I hadn't slept since Friday! Poor Dan went into the bathroom and started dry heaving from exhaustion. I was struggling with breastfeeding—it was so painful—and I could barely keep my eyes open. But napping was impossible with the number of hospital staff coming in and out of my hospital room. I sent Dan home so he could get some uninterrupted sleep.

By that evening, I was desperate to rest, as it had been 72 hours since I'd closed my eyes. The night nurse offered to take my baby away so I could have some time to sleep. I agreed, but asked her not to give Clara any formula as we were still working hard to establish breastfeeding.

When the nurse brought her back a few hours later, I was disheartened to see that Clara was spitting up formula.

After one more busy day of sleeplessness and constant visitors and staff coming in and out of my room, I was discharged the next afternoon.

Looking back on what happened, some of my story might seem somewhat nightmarish. But part of you might be thinking that what I experienced wasn't *that* bad. I had a healthy baby, right? I gave birth vaginally and stayed in one piece—I didn't have major abdominal surgery, like one-third of American women do when giving birth. I didn't even experience any major tears when the baby came out! Although the staff put pressure on me to follow certain policies and recommendations, they were always friendly and polite. So, what was off about this situation and why does it matter?

Even today, it's hard for me to put my finger on it. But if I had to sum it up, I think there were quite a few wrong things that happened at my daughter's birth. First, my baby and I were treated like we were sick, even though we were healthy all along. Second, I was coerced to have specific interventions instead of being given true alternatives and then being supported in my choices. Third, you might have noticed that I was never offered any comfort measures or support from my nurses other than an epidural. No tub, no shower, no positioning, no massage, no ability to walk around, no breastfeeding support. Dan and I were left alone for most of our labor—I was in pain in a cold, clinical place, with no idea of what was going to happen next.

Fourth, I experienced a lot of pressure to receive unnecessary interventions that caused bad things to happen down the line. For example, I was made to lie on my back, which slowed down labor, increased my pain, and may have prevented my baby from getting into an optimal position for birth. That led to the use of Pitocin® and an epidural, which led to a long pushing phase and a vacuum-assisted birth, and, ultimately, hours of separation between me and my baby during the most important bonding time humans experience in their lifetimes. The domino effect of one-intervention-leading-to-another actually has a name among professionals in the childbirth field: the cascade of interventions.

I tell this story of my first daughter's birth because I'm not alone. When I share this story with others, about half the time, the person I'm telling the story to starts crying. Why are they crying? Because they identify with my story. But why are they crying, even if it's been years—sometimes decades—after giving birth? Because what happens in birth stays with you the rest of your life. Those feelings never leave, especially the distress at being separated from your newborn.

I always knew something was wrong with how tears welled in my eyes when I thought about my separation from Clara. But I never knew why! Why on earth would I cry when I remembered her birth, the day that should've been the most joyful of my life?

It wasn't until years later, when I met Dr. Cheryl Beck, a world-renowned researcher on birth trauma and postpartum mood disorders, and I shared my birth story with her, that I finally received the answer I was searching for. "Rebecca," she said, her eyes locked with mine. "That was birth trauma."

Birth trauma[8] is defined as a birth event with actual or threatened serious injury or death *or* when the person giving birth feels they have been stripped of their dignity or treated inhumanely. Birth trauma is estimated to occur in 33% to 45% of all births in the U.S. and Australia. These numbers are astoundingly high, and explain why it's so common to hear "horror stories" about childbirth from family and friends. Women who experience birth trauma often describe cold, unsupportive, or degrading and inhumane care. Their care providers don't communicate with them—they may talk over them as if they're not there. The woman may fear for their safety or that of their baby, especially if they're told they must comply "so we can keep your baby safe." And in the end, their experience is almost never validated. Everyone tells them, "But you have a healthy baby."

I was fortunate in that I did not develop any major psychological ramifications from my birth trauma. Some people who experience birth trauma will go on to develop PTSD—post-traumatic stress disorder. You're more likely to develop PTSD after a traumatic birth experience if you have a history of anxiety, depression, or trauma, or if you experienced medical complications such as Cesarean or a postpartum hemorrhage. People who are survivors of sexual assault are at especially high risk for PTSD after birth trauma. This is because many abuse survivors are exposed to traumatic triggers during labor, such as during vaginal exams.

On the opposite end of the spectrum from birth trauma, I learned that researchers have found that some people feel incredibly satisfied and empowered after giving birth. Some people, in fact, are so excited by their birth experiences that they make a career out of birth—going into nursing, midwifery, or doula work.

Learning this fact, that some people felt empowered by giving birth, made me curious. What's the difference between a scary, traumatic birth, and an empowering, satisfying one? Is it luck? Is it the presence or absence of complications? Or is it something else?

The answer is surprisingly simple. In one review of 137 studies on birth satisfaction, researchers found that the factors that most influence birth satisfaction include whether or not your expectations were met, whether or not you felt involved in decision-making, and how you were treated by your care providers.[9]

I didn't have very high expectations for this birth. I wanted to get through it without having surgery, and I did, so in that respect, I was satisfied. I actually wrote in my journal a few weeks after, "I'm so happy with our birth, and I wouldn't have had it go any other way." But I was still so blind. I didn't know how good birth *could* be. I didn't know what it was like to have a childbirth care team focused on empowering me while also helping keep me and my baby safe. If I had known in that moment what I was missing out on, I might have been even more traumatized. But as it was, I was still pretty naïve.

I did know, though, that my baby and I should have been given time to bond and get to know each other. That it was wrong for the staff to separate us. Why did they do that? Didn't they realize the harm they could cause? Why were they so flippant about keeping Clara away from me during the first hours of her life? Why did they think it wasn't a big deal?

I didn't know the answers to all of these "why" questions. All I knew was that I left birth feeling exhausted and disempowered, and I started parenthood that way as well.

Chapter Two

EVIDENCE

THE NEXT TWO WEEKS after giving birth were a blur. I was indescribably tired from labor and birth and from the sleepless days and nights I spent caring for a newborn. I felt like I'd been run over by a truck from pushing for three hours—every muscle in my body hurt from the strain. Also, my legs and ankles that had felt like elephant legs during labor were now elephant legs in real life! That's because they were swollen from the large amount of IV fluids I'd received during my long labor.

Breastfeeding was difficult, mainly because I had additional swelling in my breasts that was incredibly painful, but also because the hospital staff had never taught me how to latch my baby properly. There was no one to call for help. My mom didn't live nearby, and none of my local friends had given birth yet, much less knew how to breastfeed.

Crying and desperate, I searched online for "breastfeeding support" and found something called La Leche League, a group that has free, regular support meetings for new moms. I dragged myself out of my house (you cannot even imagine what goes into leaving the house with a newborn baby!) and sat on the floor next to another mom, who was also holding her two-week-old baby. We were both in tears. Me, from the pain and frustration I was experiencing, her, from her mother-in-law who kept trying to give the baby formula.

But the support we received there was the turning point for me (and, as I found out a year later when I ran into that same mom at a local swimming pool, it was the turning point for her, as well!). I finally had someone show me how to correctly latch my baby, eliminating the pain I'd had for two weeks now. They also taught me how to handle a problem I'd been having with an over-abundance of milk.

From that point on, I started getting the hang of things and my world changed. Motherhood actually became fun! I thoroughly enjoyed being a mom and getting to know my precious little daughter. I stopped by my university, where I worked as a PhD student, and my fellow students, research team members, and professors oohed and ahhed over my baby. One of my mentors mentioned that I had a "new mom glow." Funny how a little bit of support and teaching tipped me from desperation into bliss. If I hadn't gone to that La Leche League meeting, my next chance to get support wouldn't have been for another month. In the U.S., women typically don't get checked by any sort of health care provider until six weeks postpartum. It wouldn't be until ten years after my giving birth to Clara that the professional association for obstetricians in the U.S., the American Congress of Obstetricians and Gynecologists, would call for the first postpartum visit to take place in the first three weeks after giving birth.[10]

I don't like to think what would have happened had I not been able to find postpartum support on my own.

A year and a half later, in the spring of 2010, I walked across a commencement stage, and my faculty mentor draped a doctoral hood over my shoulders. Dan, Clara, and our families were in the audience, cheering me on. While caring for an infant, I'd managed to complete my dissertation and earn a PhD in Nursing! In my PhD program, which is essentially a research program, I had learned how to read and write research papers and conduct clinical research in health care—even carrying out my own randomized, controlled trial and publishing four peer-reviewed journal articles prior to graduation.

I accepted a job to be an assistant professor in the same nursing program where I had earned my master's and doctorate. Being a professor had always been my dream job and I was thrilled! I couldn't wait to work full time with nursing students and to continue conducting clinical research. By this point, I already knew that my life's mission was to make an impact in other people's lives, and what better way to do this than to educate the next generation of nurses, and to carry out research that influences patient care?

As I settled into my new faculty position, I started thinking about my experience giving birth. It had been nearly two years since Clara was born, but it seemed like I was finally ready to process—truly process—everything that had been done to me in the hospital. Through reading books and watching documentaries, I began to realize that my story was a classic example of the "standard" or "routine" care that happens in a lot of hospitals. I mulled over what I had gone through—the unnecessary pain and frustration. The separation. The pressure and coercion. The nurse's refusal to let me walk to the bathroom. I started questioning *everything*.

Dan and I had hoped to add to our family around this time, but unfortunately, not only was it difficult to get pregnant, but both times I did get pregnant, I miscarried. As a result, I felt heartbroken, lonely, and depressed. I remember riding my bike to the university and crying a week after I miscarried for the second time. Would that baby have been a boy or girl? I would never know. The losses haunted me.

But the miscarriages also gave me extra time to think, and read, and plan. While I mourned the loss of my pregnancies and waited and waited for another pregnancy to finally stick, I wondered . . . what was the *evidence* for everything that was done to me in the hospital when Clara was born?

Evidence based care is defined as using research to help inform medical decision-making, considering the health care worker's expertise and the patient's values, goals, and preferences. In the 1990s, the founders of evidence based medicine,[11] Dr. David Sackett, Dr. Gordan Guyatt, and others, wrote that evidence based care is a three-legged stool, made up of

1. Research evidence
2. A provider who is trained in how to help you interpret evidence, and
3. Care that is tailored to your own values, goals, and preferences.

Now, I'm sure many people believe this is how care is already delivered. But the truth is, a good portion of health care—including care during childbirth—is still based on long-standing tradition and doctors' opinions, as well as financial incentives, financial disincentives, and fears of liability. Believe it or not, research is usually more of an afterthought rather than a foundation for current medical practice. Researchers have found that it takes, on average, 15 to 20 years after something is proven in medical research before it becomes used routinely in hospitals.[12] This time lapse even has a well-known name—the "evidence-practice gap."

One key aspect of my new job was the fact that I was totally immersed in the concept of "evidence based care." It was considered a primary element of being a nurse, and as faculty, we were continually teaching our nursing students how to use research evidence in how they cared for patients. So, while I waited to get pregnant again, I decided to look up the research and figure out whether or not my care with Clara had been evidence based. I started by making a bullet-point list of everything that had happened to me during Clara's birth, and dug up the research on each topic.

As I read the research, I was shocked to find that almost everything that was done to me during my birth had already been proven by research evidence to be either not helpful or actually harmful to healthy people who are giving birth! Here's what I discovered:

Not allowed to eat or drink fluids during labor. This practice originated in the 1940s and continues because many doctors and anesthesiologists believe it is necessary to fast during labor. But research has shown that eating and drinking during labor is safe and makes women much more satisfied with their birth.[13] Researchers have concluded that people have the right to decide if they would like to eat or drink during labor. There was no scientific basis for making me fast for a whole day and night while my body was essentially running a marathon. In fact, I discovered that, unlike in the U.S., some practitioners in other parts of the world actually encourage women to eat and drink because it's assumed you'll need the energy for birth!

Not allowed out of bed during labor. Evidence shows that this practice is harmful.[14] Researchers have carried out large trials where they randomly assign people to be in upright positions or lying down during labor. They found that being restricted to bed leads to longer, more painful labors, and increases your chances of requesting an epidural or giving birth by Cesarean. Babies born to mothers who labored in bed-lying positions are also more likely to be admitted to the newborn intensive care unit.

The nurses insisted I stay in bed because my water had broken, and that sitting or standing upright could cause a rare emergency called cord prolapse, when the baby's cord could drop down below the baby's head. I looked up the research on that situation as well. Turns out, there is no evidence showing that you're more likely to have cord prolapse just because your water broke at the start of labor.[15] I had been restricted to bed and exposed to the risks of bed rest for no good reason.

Intravenous fluids during labor. I wasn't allowed to drink liquids, so I was hooked up to fluids that dripped into a vein in my arm. But evidence shows that, first of all, you shouldn't deny people oral fluids during labor.[13] Second of all, when you are free to eat and drink oral fluids, intravenous fluids aren't always needed, since most of the time you can give yourself whatever hydration and nutrition you need.[16] Also, a few studies that have started to look at the effects of IV fluids on breastfeeding found that excess amounts of these fluids during birth can cause painful breast swelling in the mother[17] and an artificial weight drop in the baby.[18, 19, 20] This explained my difficulty with breastfeeding! The painful tissue swelling in my arms, legs, and breasts was related to too high a volume of fluids pumped into my body during labor.

Continuous fetal monitoring. One of the first things the nurse did was hook me up to an electronic monitor to track my baby's heart rate. Amazingly, large randomized trials have shown that this type of monitoring is not very good at getting accurate information about what's happening with the baby. Overall, it has not been shown to reduce the rate of stillbirth or newborn death, while it increases the chance that the mother will have a Cesarean.[21]

Put another way, hooking someone up to an electronic fetal monitor increases risks to the mother without significantly improving safety for the baby, other than reducing the risk of rare seizure events (from about one seizure in 325 births without continuous monitoring to one in 650 births with continuous monitoring).

A more evidence based option, which is rarely used, is for nurses or providers to hold a small handheld Doppler or fetal stethoscope to your abdomen and listen to the baby's heart rate at prescribed intervals. This method, sometimes called "hands-on listening" or "intermittent auscultation," also has the benefit of making sure the mother is still able to move around. In contrast, the electronic monitor requires you to stay in bed all or most of the time. Although there are "mobile" monitors on the market today, there is very little research on mobile monitors, and women tell me that hospital staff often make them lie still in bed even with a mobile monitor so staff can get a better reading on the baby.

Pitocin® to speed up labor, also called Pitocin® augmentation. Research has shown that when people are in labor spontaneously (meaning they weren't induced with medication), Pitocin® or synthetic oxytocin, the drug I reluctantly agreed to after lots of pressure, may shorten labor by an average of two hours, but not reduce my risk of having a Cesarean.[22] I learned that, had I instead been encouraged to walk around and be upright, it likely would have shortened labor by an average of about one and a half hours *and* significantly reduced the risk of having a Cesarean.[14] Randomized trials have also demonstrated that if you're a first-time mother with a slow labor, getting into a warm tub of water can reduce your need for augmentation with Pitocin® and/or an amniotomy (where the care provider breaks your water), reduce pain, and increase satisfaction, without increasing the length of labor.[23]

I also learned that Pitocin® is considered a high-alert drug, meaning that there's a high risk of harm if a health care worker happened to make an error while administering the drug.[24] Because of this, Pitocin® should be used with care—only when there is a medical need that outweighs the risks of using it. I was still in early labor when Pitocin® was suggested to me, and I now know that it's normal for early labor to last a long time in a first-time mom whose water broke before the start of regular contractions at term. Half of people in this situation are in early labor for less than 17 hours and half are in early labor even longer.[25] Yet I was not offered any alternatives to speed up labor, and I was told that I was experiencing something "abnormal" that needed a medication to fix.

Frequent vaginal exams. One of the first things done to me when I got to the hospital was "checking" my cervix during a vaginal exam. For people whose water broke at the start of labor, like me, the number of vaginal exams you have during labor is one of the most important risk factors for developing an infection called chorioamnionitis.

Vaginal exams can lead to chorioamnionitis in someone whose water is broken because the staff member's gloved fingers (even though the gloves are "sterile!") push bacteria from the bottom of the vagina up to the cervix as they conduct the exam. Research has shown that vaginal exams nearly double the number of types of bacteria at the cervix.[26] In one large trial of people whose water had broken, the researchers compared people who had two or fewer vaginal exams to everyone else.[25,27] They found that women who had three to four vaginal exams had two times the odds of developing chorioamnionitis, those who had five to six exams had 2.6 times the odds of getting the infection, those who had seven to eight vaginal exams had 3.8 times the odds, and those who had more than eight exams had five times the odds.

I'm not sure how many vaginal exams I had after my water broke at the onset of labor. It was at least five or six. Because of the hospital staff's desire to keep close tabs on my dilation, they had more than doubled my risk of developing an infection.

Now, if my water hadn't broken at the start of labor, there would be less risk of infection with the vaginal exams because intact membranes help protect you from infection. Still, whether or not your water has broken, vaginal exams can be highly uncomfortable—in fact, for me they were extremely painful—and I would have liked to avoid them if possible. I heard later on, from clinicians who worked at my university's hospital, that the culture there was to check a laboring woman's cervix every two hours if their water hadn't broken, and less frequently if their water had broken. Clinicians were under a lot of pressure to write those every-two-hour exam results on a big whiteboard at the nurse's station. I couldn't find any research that showed benefits to frequent vaginal exams during labor. It turns out that this extremely common practice is based on tradition and routine, not on evidence.[28]

Epidural for managing discomfort. Epidurals are highly effective at helping manage discomfort during labor.[29] Another benefit is that they can help you rest, relax, and get some sleep during labor, especially if you've been in labor for a long time. There is also some evidence that severe, untreated pain (when someone is suffering, not coping with labor) can lead to a higher maternal stress response and decreased blood flow to the baby. Effective pain management may reduce maternal stress reactions and improve blood supply to the baby.[30]

However, epidurals do come with potential side effects,[29] such as the risk of a drop in your blood pressure (which can then drop the baby's heart rate), problems passing urine, and fever. As I experienced firsthand, epidurals can lead to being unable to move or feel sensation for a period of time after the birth (also called a motor block) and can increase the need for a vacuum or forceps birth. Rare but potentially severe side effects include long-lasting headache and nerve damage after the injection. I was informed of all these benefits and risks, so that part of my care was evidence based.

But there are plenty of other, less risky comfort measures that I was not offered. For example, getting in a warm tub of water doesn't carry any of the risks of an epidural, but can be very effective for increasing comfort.[31] Movement has been shown to drastically increase comfort during labor,[14] especially when it's combined with the use of an exercise "birth ball."[32] A large survey of mothers who gave birth in U.S. hospitals found that mothers rated laboring in a tub, pool, or shower and laboring with a birth ball as providing even more effective pain relief than opioids.[33] Some other non-pharmacologic comfort measures that have been shown by research to be beneficial include acupressure,[34] aromatherapy,[35,36] massage,[37] and music.[38,39] I was not educated about any of these comfort measures in my hospital childbirth class, and while I was in labor, zero non-pharmacologic comfort measures were offered to me—in fact, movement was explicitly forbidden.

Also, for me, the birth environment was incredibly stressful and unsupportive, which may have increased my discomfort! In one study with 600 mothers, researchers measured pain intensity during labor, then interviewed mothers afterward about environmental stressors.[40] The mothers reported stressors such as crowded and noisy birthing rooms and restrictions on movement and fluid intake. The researchers concluded that environmental stressors can aggravate pain and anxiety levels during labor. Other researchers have found that loud noises during labor increase fear, which can make a person more sensitive to pain.[41] The temperature of the room, the brightness of light in the room, and the feeling of being observed can also stimulate the brain to release stress hormones.[42] It's important for care providers to help women cope with labor by providing privacy, avoiding unnecessary procedures or restrictions that may cause stress or tension, and working to identify sources of disturbances and removing them.

Looking back, I would have preferred to have a birth environment in which I felt supported and private. The crowds, lack of privacy, and restrictions on my eating, drinking, and movement were unnecessary stressors that increased my anxiety and discomfort. I also would have liked to start out using non-medical comfort measures, and then switched to an epidural only if the non-medical approaches were not helpful enough.

Continuous labor support. Labor support is defined as the therapeutic presence of another person, and includes physical support, emotional support, information, and advocacy.[43] Surprisingly, most nurses have no training in "hands-on" labor support skills—it's not taught in most nursing schools, nor in most hospital orientations for new nurses. Nurses also have other patients and responsibilities, and hospital culture sometimes frowns on nurses spending too much time with patients. For whatever reason, I did not receive labor support from my nurses. It was a major gap in my care.

However, doulas are an option for filling that gap! A doula is a companion who supports someone during labor and birth. Birth doulas are trained to provide continuous, one-on-one care, as well as information, advocacy, physical support, and emotional support to both the birthing person and their partner. Their essential role is to support you, no matter what decisions you make or how you give birth.

In one of the most important studies on doulas, researchers randomly assigned 420 first-time mothers to only receive support from their partner, or to care that also included a professional doula.[44] The results showed a huge improvement in outcomes for women who had both a partner and a doula, compared to having a partner alone. The Cesarean rate for first-time mothers was 13% in the group with a partner and a doula and 25% in the group with a partner only. Fewer women in the doula group required an epidural compared to those without a doula, and 100% of people in this study who had a doula rated their experience as positive or very positive.

My obstetrician and the educator in my hospital childbirth class never encouraged me to hire a doula, and my hospital did not provide one. I had asked Dan about the possibility of a doula, but he thought it would be weird to have a "stranger" in the room when I was giving birth. Little did we know that our room would be packed to the brim with strangers as the baby was emerging. In retrospect, the doula would've been one of the only people in the room we knew ahead of time.

Water immersion during birth. I knew that laboring in water was safe, but what about water birth, defined as remaining in the water during the pushing phase and birth of the baby? Was that a safe option? I found that there have been many observational studies on water birth (with more than 31,000 water births studied), and a few randomized trials.[45, 46] The available research showed both potential benefits and risks with water birth. Benefits include lower levels of pain and higher levels of satisfaction, as well as fewer interventions and less use of medication for pain relief.

In terms of the maternal risks, recent research has shown a higher rate of mild tears from water birth in homes and birth centers.[47] However, in hospital settings, researchers have found that water birth is associated with lower rates of severe tears and much lower rates of episiotomy (an episiotomy is a traumatic cut of the skin between the vagina and rectum).[45]

Large observational studies have not shown any increase in the risk of newborn death or any other bad health outcome for newborns, including neonatal intensive care admissions, low Apgar scores, breathing difficulty, need for resuscitation, or infections.[46]

There have been some case studies of bad outcomes for newborns. There have been several reports of water aspiration,[48, 49] when the newborn breathed in water before they were lifted out of the tub, but this side effect has not been observed in observational studies since 1999,[50] and almost all of the infants in the individual case reports made a complete recovery. Also, although large studies have not seen any increase in the risk of infection, there have been several individual reports of newborn infection after water birth.[48, 51, 52] Practice guidelines state that this rare risk can be lowered even further by using pools that are easy to disinfect, filling tubs closer to the time of the birth (i.e., not letting the water stand for a long time), and, if giving birth in a hospital, performing regular bacterial tests on the water supply, hoses, and birthing tubs.[53]

Based on the evidence, it seemed to me that water birth was a reasonable option, provided that I understood the benefits and risks and made an informed choice. I decided that I would play it by ear, and consider staying in a warm tub for the birth of my next baby.

Pushing positions. One of the least effective pushing positions is lying on your back or semi-sitting in bed. This makes the sacrum (or tailbone) inflexible, which makes it harder for your baby to exit your body, especially with gravity working against both of you. Research has shown that when people without epidurals get in upright birthing positions—such as squatting, hands and knees, standing, or kneeling—that they're much less likely to get an episiotomy, less likely to give birth with vacuum or forceps, and the pushing phase is shortened.[54] The side-lying position is helpful for women with epidurals. Giving birth in a supported side-lying position with an epidural has been shown to reduce the length of the active pushing phase and make it less likely that the mother will have an episiotomy or give birth with vacuum or forceps.[55] I was made to lie on my back the whole time, and nobody ever suggested that I push on my side.

Coached pushing. The intense yelling at me to hold my breath and push (also known as "purple pushing" because sometimes your face turns purple from holding your breath) was also not necessary; there is no evidence that coached pushing provides any benefits over spontaneous pushing (often called "mother-directed pushing") for women with or without epidurals.[56] So, in the absence of evidence showing firm benefits to either method of pushing (coached vs. mother-directed), care should be individualized to the birthing person's preference, comfort, and unique circumstances. I was never asked about my preferences for pushing.

Giving me time to push. One aspect of my care that was evidence based was the fact that my provider gave me adequate time to push my baby out. Large research studies show that for first-time mothers, especially those with epidurals, pushing may take hours![57, 58] In fact, it is an evidence based option for a first-time mother with an epidural to consider pushing for four or more hours, as long as mother and baby are doing well and making progress.[59] The fact that my provider diagnosed improper positioning of my baby and used her hands to adjust the baby's position has also been shown by evidence to help prevent Cesareans.[60] However, my baby's improper positioning may have been caused by the fact that I was instructed to labor on my back for 24 hours. This could have been a preventable complication—and an avoidable procedure that caused me stress and pain.

Early cord clamping. Something that I didn't notice at the time, but I know happened to Clara, was that they immediately clamped her umbilical cord after she was born. Early cord clamping became widespread in the 1960s, and is generally defined as clamping the umbilical cord within 30 to 60 seconds of birth.[61] Many parents don't realize there's a difference between "clamping" and "cutting" the cord—the clamp stops the blood flow from the placenta to the baby (and is usually done immediately by hospital staff, with a clamp), and the cutting is done later on (often by the partner, with scissors).

During labor and birth, one-third of the baby's blood is flowing through the placenta at any one time.[62] When hospital staff immediately clamp the cord, this means that 30% of the baby's blood volume is left behind in the placenta—and the baby only receives 70% of their own blood at birth! In contrast, if you leave the cord unclamped for a longer period of time, the baby will get 80% of their blood within 60 seconds, and 87% within 3 to 5 minutes. Babies *need* their blood—this blood helps with the fetal transition to life outside the womb. The blood that is transfusing from the placenta to the baby is rich in millions of stem cells, as well as iron, which is used to make hemoglobin. Randomized trials have found that babies whose cords are unclamped for longer periods of time have higher hemoglobin levels in the first year of life.[63] Researchers have looked at brain scans (MRIs) of infants who were randomly assigned to early or delayed cord clamping at birth and found increased brain development among the babies who received delayed clamping.[64] So, it is thought that this may improve long-term brain development in your child!

Delaying cord clamping has been shown to be so beneficial, in so many studies, that some researchers have said that there are important ethical concerns to consider before doing any more randomized trials on this subject.[55] But, at many hospitals in the U.S., early cord clamping is still routine practice! Parents may write down "delayed cord clamping" on their birth plan, but the nurses or doctors may do early cord clamping anyway, just because it's what they're used to doing. I've heard accounts of parents asking for delayed cord clamping, and physicians saying things like, "I don't delay past one minute because it's dangerous! The baby would receive too much blood." Hospital staff may also believe that delayed cord clamping increases the risk of jaundice, a yellowing of the baby's skin and eyes from the breakdown of red blood cells. While it's true that a 2013 Cochrane meta-analysis[65] found more use of light therapy to treat jaundice with delayed cord clamping (4.4%) versus early cord clamping (2.7%), this finding is based mostly on one large, unpublished dissertation study,[66] and the final conclusion of the Cochrane review was still that delayed cord clamping is beneficial. A different systematic review published in the Journal of the American Medical Association (JAMA) did not include this unpublished study, and they did not find any relationship between jaundice and delayed cord clamping.[67] None of the published randomized controlled trials on term infants have shown an increase in jaundice with delayed cord clamping.[68]

Separation from my baby. Without even looking at the evidence, I was pretty sure there's no way research would support separation of mothers and babies. But I looked it up anyway. I was right!

Separating mothers from newborn babies is extremely harmful—it's a practice that is unique to the 20th and 21st centuries and is a complete break from human history.[69] Evidence shows that the best care for mothers and babies is to provide them with uninterrupted skin-to-skin contact during the first hour or two of life, and to intermittently continue that skin-to-skin contact over the next days and weeks.[70] Skin-to-skin care (also called kangaroo care) is a natural process that involves giving a naked newborn to their mother to lie on her bare chest while covering the infant with blankets to keep them dry and warm.

As a side note, placing a baby on top of the mother's gown or on top of a towel does *not* count as skin-to-skin—it is the actual skin contact that allows hormones between the mom and baby to "communicate" with each other. To this day, it drives me crazy when I see nurses throw a towel on top of the mother's chest and abdomen so that the baby's skin won't touch the mother's skin. The skin touching part is the whole point of doing skin-to-skin care!

Babies who are held skin-to-skin with their mothers have lower stress levels, better success with breastfeeding, and more stable blood sugar, breathing, heart rate, and oxygen levels.[71]

By contrast, when babies are separated from their mothers, not only are they less able to breastfeed and have more trouble with their vital signs, but they are also twelve times more likely to cry (separation distresses babies), and their mothers are more likely to experience anxiety and breast engorgement (painful, swollen breasts) in the days after birth. My daughter and I experienced many of these side effects from being separated unnecessarily.

I also found one randomized trial, out of Russia, about the long-term effects of temporarily separating mothers and newborns after birth.[72] In this study, all babies were separated from their mothers for the first 25 minutes of life for "mandatory" routine care. Then, half the babies were returned to their mothers' arms for skin-to-skin care. The other half were tightly swaddled and kept separate from their mothers for two hours. The babies were filmed playing with their mothers one year later, and researchers who were blinded to group assignments analyzed the films. The results showed that the one-year-old infants who had been separated from their mothers at birth for two hours were more irritable, impulsive, and had trouble self-regulating. The mothers who were separated were less responsive to their infants, and showed less reciprocity and mutuality—meaning they were less enthusiastic and more likely to have a flat affect when interacting with their child.

All I can say is, I'm glad human beings are resilient. Clara and I became very bonded despite our separation, but we can't ever know what life would have been like if we'd been kept together during those crucial first hours.

I'm not sure how you feel right now, but after uncovering all this information, I was beginning to feel a bit betrayed by the system. How could it be that an institution that so valued and proclaimed support for "evidence based medicine" and "evidence based nursing" was delivering a very different type of care in their birthing unit?

As I read through the research, I became more and more upset that the care I had received in a modern academic hospital was based more on tradition and routines rather than best evidence. What's more, I found out that the type of care I had received was "routine" all across the U.S.—and that model has been copied in places all over the world!

When I got pregnant again, I wanted my next birth to be different. I wanted my baby's birth to be evidence based.

Chapter Three

DISCOVERY

A S SOON AS I GOT MY NEXT positive pregnancy test, I sat down and made a "wish list" of the type of care I wanted to have with this baby's birth:

- Freedom to eat and drink
- Freedom to move around
- Continuous support during labor
- Labor (and possibly give birth) in a warm tub of water
- Monitoring the baby during labor with a handheld device (aka intermittent auscultation) instead of the electronic fetal monitor
- No IV fluids unless medically necessary
- Few or no vaginal exams
- Pushing and giving birth in an upright position
- Keeping my baby with me after birth—no separation
- Rest and relaxation (naps and sleep during early labor and after the birth)
- Lots of skin-to-skin care

This list seemed wonderful to me. The only problem was, how was I supposed to get these things when my hospital was not willing to support everything on this list?

Also, not only did I want to be free from unnecessary interventions, I wanted to be free from *coercion and pressure* to have unnecessary interventions. I didn't want to have to *fight* during labor. This was important to me for several reasons. First, I had experienced firsthand how disturbing it was to have people continually trying to pressure you into things during labor—it's distracting and stressful. Stress during labor can activate your *sympathetic nervous system*, or fight/flight response, which is thought to slow down labor.[73] Second, I am a people pleaser. It scares me that I might make people upset or angry with me because of my choices. One of my greatest fears is to be disliked by people I have to work with in a close setting.

Remember how obedient I wanted to be in that first birth? Well, there's a reason for that. I've been burned in the past by people who were upset by the decisions I've made. In particular, in high school, I lost nearly all of my close friends except two—my lifelong best friend Sarah and my sister Shannon—after I spoke up when I thought something my other friends were doing was wrong. My words, and the rejection I experienced as a result, came at a heavy cost. I spent the rest of my senior year eating my lunch alone in a stairwell.

Ever since that humiliating experience, I've been very careful about what I speak up about, weighing the consequences of my words. With every sentence, I worry, "Will this make someone my enemy? Will they stop being my friend?" I was always an introvert, but after that experience, I became even more private, and to this day, I've kept my social group small. I only confide in a few people whom I could truly trust, and they have to be people whose principles—kindness, fairness, honesty—match my own. For many years, that circle included only my parents, Shannon, and Sarah. It eventually widened to include Dan, and a few more people you'll meet later on.

Given my first birth story, and my fear of upsetting people, it only made sense that I should surround myself at my birth with people who supported my decisions wholeheartedly. But like I said earlier, who could support me? I'd already seen what kind of pressure I faced to follow all the hospital polices, and what happened when I tried to refuse one routine procedure (Pitocin®).

In fact, at my university's hospital, it was not realistic for me to expect to get most of the items on my wish list. The only exception was skin-to-skin, since by the time I was due with my second baby, my hospital had started doing skin-to-skin care as part of their journey toward becoming Baby-Friendly® (an international designation awarded to hospitals that foster practices that support breastfeeding).

So here I was a few years after my first baby was born, wanting evidence based care, and not sure what to do. I eventually realized that I needed to find someone *already practicing evidence based care* as part of their normal routine.

I don't remember how or when I realized that midwives might be the solution to my problem, but when I discovered midwives, it was like the skies opened up and I awoke to a whole new world. I was not alone in the fact that I did not know what a midwife was beforehand. Today, most college students I teach have no idea what a midwife actually does or is trained to do. When I ask them to write down the first word that comes to their mind when I say "midwife" almost all of the students leave their paper blank. They can't write something down in association with the word midwife because they literally do not know what to think about midwives. It is not part of their life story.

So, what did I discover?

The word "midwife" comes from the Middle English words "mid" (with) and "wife" (woman), which, combined, means *with woman*. Midwives are practiced in the art and science of being with women and supporting them in pregnancy and birth. They are experts in helping women use their own bodies to give birth safely, and they can handle most emergencies short of surgery. Today, some people hire a midwife if they're interested in having a physiologic birth without an epidural. But midwives who work in hospital settings use epidurals as desired with their clients, as well. Midwives believe strongly in your autonomy, and they support you in whatever choices you make.[74]

Throughout most of human history, childbirth was a female-led, community-oriented activity; "midwives" often meant local women who had experience giving birth themselves and who might feel called to help other women—with or without special training or payment for their services. Over time, midwifery developed as a formal profession of women helping other women through this major life event, passing on wisdom, training, and knowledge about birth to each other—through formal education programs, apprenticeship, or, usually, both.

Most people don't realize that midwifery existed long before medicine. When the medical specialty of obstetrics was developed a few hundred years ago—exclusively by men at the time—pregnancy was viewed as a disease and, in many ways, birth was something to be feared and managed. But before the onset of modern medicine, before the last few hundred years, midwives were the *exclusive* birth attendants around the world. Each culture had their own midwives—Hebrew midwives played an important role in the Bible; legendary Black "granny" or "grand" midwives brought their knowledge from West Africa to the U.S., attending the births of most Black and White women in the Old South; European midwives passed their considerable wisdom down through the generations and across the ocean via the many midwives who immigrated to the U.S. from the 1600s through the 1900s; from the 1800s on, most of them were trained in European professional midwifery schools. Indigenous midwives of the Americas attended births of their community members before the medicalization of birth and they continue to work today to preserve and advance traditional midwifery.[74,75]

Despite their role in supporting women and babies in the process of birth throughout all of history and pre-history, midwives are now only present at 10% of births in the U.S.[76] Furthermore, the Black Grand Midwives are gone, and the vast majority of midwives left are White, with very few women of color working in the midwifery profession.[77]

What happened? Where did the midwives go?

The answer is a tragic story mixed up with both sexism and racism. In the year 1900 in the U.S., more than 95% of all births occurred at home. About 50% of all births were attended by midwives, and 50% were attended by physicians, many of whom were general practitioners.[78] The midwife-attended birth rate was even higher among ethnic minorities and women in rural areas. In 1918, for example, midwives still attended 86% of births to Italian-American immigrants in Chicago, and in 1922, granny midwives attended 85% of the births to women in rural Kentucky. As late as 1936, midwives attended 42% of all Georgia births.[79]

Around this time, obstetricians in the burgeoning American Medical Association began realizing that childbirth could be a huge market for them. And they were right! Today, pregnancy, childbirth, and newborn care are by far the most common reasons for hospitalizations—making up about 23% of all U.S. hospital stays.[80] But before obstetricians could move in and take over the market, they had to figure out how to get rid of the competition.[74, 75]

Sadly, eliminating midwives in the U.S. was pretty easy. In the early 1900s, all midwives were female, and many were black- or brown-skinned, or immigrants. They did not share the same language, nor culture, and they often did not even know of the others' existence. The midwives were unable to form a national association or coalition that might have supported them and established midwifery as a profession early on—as it already was in European countries, where midwives have always, and still today, attend the vast majority of births. Despite their considerable skills, and the fact that many were professionally educated in Europe, most midwives were stereotyped as "uneducated." Physicians were aghast that women might work as midwives—it was thought that women were mentally unfit to make decisions about themselves or others.

White men, and White male physicians specifically, held enormous power politically, financially, and socially. This left midwives at a huge disadvantage—even though midwives were providing safer care and had lower maternal mortality rates than physicians.[74, 75]

Obstetricians and allied medical and public health professionals devised a three-pronged approach to take over the childbirth market. First, they launched a national propaganda campaign that played on popular racist and sexist sentiments to convince the public that female midwives were dirty, foreign, and ignorant. With these ideas planted, wealthy women began to seek out the care of obstetricians in hospitals, and lower-income women eventually followed suit. Second, physicians began systematically changing state and local laws to outlaw midwifery, or, if it couldn't be forbidden, to tightly restrict midwifery practice and require midwives to be "supervised" by physicians. Third, obstetricians sought to lower the public's perception of general practitioners, or family doctors, so that women would only seek out obstetricians for maternity care. By eliminating midwives and family doctors from the childbirth scene, obstetricians solidified their monopoly on deliveries. The monopoly also ensured that obstetricians had enough delivery "cases" to train medical students and residents in their specialty, continuing their dominance of the market.[74,75]

Not only was the physicians' campaign successful in either eliminating or tightly regulating midwifery care across the nation, physicians ensured that most of the remaining midwives would be White. At first, the Southern Black "granny" midwives, who cared for most of the women in the Old South, were given licenses to practice by their states. But within a few years, their licenses were revoked, forcing them to retire or stop practicing to avoid prosecution.[74] By the 1970s, the Black Grand midwives had been almost fully eradicated from the South, and to this day, the vast majority of American midwives are White.[81]

Around the same time that obstetricians were convincing women to forsake midwives, another strange thing happened. In 1914, the periodical *McClure's Magazine* published an article called "Painless Childbirth," written by two mothers, Marguerite Tracy and Constance Leupp. The article advocated for a wonderful new method of childbirth called "Twilight Sleep," defined as giving women a mixture of morphine (for pain) and scopolamine (for sedation and amnesia) during the first stage of labor. At first, U.S. physicians were reluctant to use Twilight Sleep—they saw it as unstudied and potentially dangerous. But women demanded this pain relief option. They established a grassroots organization called the National Twilight Sleep Association, organized rallies in department stores, and garnered extensive press coverage. Despite their initial reluctance, doctors all over the country began adopting Twilight Sleep. And some obstetricians realized that they could use the marketing promise of "painless birth" to encourage more hospital births, which would hasten the decline of midwives and general practitioners, whom they saw as inferior competitors.[82]

Chances are that many women in your family experienced Twilight Sleep, because it didn't fall out of favor until the 1970s. In fact, my own mother, Carol, experienced Twilight Sleep twice when she gave birth to two of my older siblings in the 1960s. My mom was only 19 years old when she had her first baby. She had a difficult pregnancy with hyperemesis gravidarum, and she was anxious about labor and birth. She asked to be induced at 38 weeks because her husband, my dad, was scheduled to be on flight duty for the Air Force and would be out of the country for the next three months.

When my mom got to the hospital for the induction, the first thing they did was separate her from my dad at the elevator—he wasn't even allowed on the same floor. Then a nurse started the induction medications through an IV, and left my mom to labor alone in a room that had a stretcher and a clock.

The nurse came back in later and said, "Oh, you poor thing. You're so young. Do you want something for the pain?"

My mom, scared and alone, said yes.

The nurse gave my mother a cocktail of drugs. My mom has no memory of the birth after that. But she does know that they used a gas mask to give her general anesthesia during the actual delivery. They also cut an episiotomy and probably used forceps to get the baby out. And when she woke up, there was no baby in her room. The baby had been taken to the nursery, where she was kept for three days. My mom was only allowed brief, scheduled visits with her baby.

The second time my mom gave birth, about four years later, she had a similar experience. Only this time, when my mom was finally allowed to meet her baby on the second day postpartum, she discovered that my sister had black and blue bruises all over her face and head. The only reason my mom knows what happened was because there was a nurse who was a patient in the bed next to her. The nurse told my mom that the doctor used "high" forceps to pull my sister out—meaning they wrenched the baby out with forceps while she was still high up in my mother's pelvis.

There were several major problems with the Twilight Sleep that was given to many American women for more than half a century. The first problem was that it did not actually fulfill the promise of having a "painless birth." Women still felt all the pain of labor and birth! It's just that they didn't remember their suffering. Their arms and legs were tied down as they screamed and thrashed around on a "crib-bed"—at times, they were even placed in straightjackets.[82] Later, Twilight Sleep evolved to use even stronger sedative medications, as well as general anesthesia during the second stage of delivery.[83] Tragically, women sometimes died when they were overly sedated. For example, in Michigan, obstetric anesthesia was the 4th leading cause of maternal death in the 1950s. Researchers found that most of these deaths occurred when obstetric anesthesia was administered by staff who had little to no training in anesthesiology.[84] And my mother tells me that, back then, families were almost never told why mothers or babies died during childbirth.

Another major problem with Twilight Sleep was that the medications used to induce maternal sedation passed through the placenta and impacted the health of newborns. Babies usually required resuscitation after a Twilight Sleep birth, and they were too sleepy to effectively breastfeed or interact with their mothers for an entire week.[85] Mothers were also too sleepy to hold or care for their babies. Fear of germs was extremely high, so hospitals kept babies away from their mothers in central nurseries, and mothers were only permitted to see their babies a few times per day for scheduled visits. Breastfeeding was discouraged, because it was not "scientific" like formula. And husbands were only permitted to visit their wives once per day. However, postpartum visits from family, as well as the option of Twilight Sleep, were mainly limited to White women, as hospitals remained segregated and many refused admittance to Black women until well into the late 1960s.[83]

You probably think Twilight Sleep and the practices of the early-to-mid 1900s sound horrific, and they were. You also might be wondering why women fought so hard for this option! Well, in the early 1900s, the suffrage movement was in full swing. Gaining control over the pain of birth seemed like a natural step in the process towards achieving equal rights for women. But what women didn't realize is that their advocacy efforts for more control over the pain of childbirth would backfire—putting them at higher risk for death and complications, and impacting the birth options of their descendants—*you*—today.[82]

Why do I say that Twilight Sleep still impacts us today? Because some practices that originated in the era of Twilight Sleep are still around! In Chapter Two, I mentioned the practice of "not allowing" food or drink during labor. During the era of Twilight Sleep, doctors and nurses would often administer gas, or general anesthesia, during the pushing phase and vaginal delivery. Back then, they didn't have accurate ways to dose gas or protect the patient's airway. Women would sometimes vomit during the birth, and then aspirate the vomit into their lungs, leading to pneumonia and sometimes death. Although general anesthesia is never used during vaginal births today, and we have much safer ways of administering gas during the 6% of Cesareans that require it, doctors still forbid food and drink during labor in many hospitals.[86]

Data collected during the era of Twilight Sleep were also used to set a standard (called "Friedman's Curve") for how fast women should dilate during labor, leading countless women to have Cesareans for the diagnosis of "failure to progress." We now know that Friedman's Curve, calculated by Dr. Friedman in the 1950s when women were sedated or unconscious during labor,[87] cannot be applied to women of the 21st century.[88] But the diagnosis of failure to progress is still one of the most common reasons for preventable Cesareans today,[89] and Friedman's Curve appeared in medical textbooks as recently as 2010.[90]

However, perhaps one of the most harmful aspects of Twilight Sleep was that it perpetuated the myth that a delivery is a mechanical procedure, and that doctors don't have to ask permission before they do something to a patient during labor and birth. Back then, doctors and nurses would just . . . *do things.* Women were sedated or unconscious, so there was no need to get consent for anything. People giving birth were viewed as passive, dehumanized objects, and their role was to lay in bed and be delivered of a baby. As Dr. Judith Leavitt pointed out in an article about the history of Twilight Sleep, one obstetrician said that anesthesia gave "absolute control over your patient at all stages of the game . . . You are 'boss.'"[82] Believe it or not, in many places around the world, this kind of sexist attitude about women's bodies during birth is still a big problem.

Gradually, as Twilight Sleep fell out of favor, and the epidural took its place, some practices did improve. Women could now be awake and alert when their babies were born. And partners were gradually allowed into the birthing room—although, for many years, that privilege was only extended to White married women of a certain class.[83]

But here's the deal. There was no one moment where everyone stopped and said, "Hey, that Twilight Sleep thing? That was really bad. Let's take a step back, evaluate our practices, and see what we can do to humanize the birth process and provide safer, better care for moms and babies." Instead, we embarked on a painstakingly slow journey of change, in which families had to fight for every incremental improvement in care. Women had to fight for the right to have their partners by their side. They had to fight to be able to breastfeed and keep their babies with them after the birth. It took decades for rates of episiotomy and forceps use to decrease. And today, vestiges of the medicalized culture of Twilight Sleep remain stubbornly intact in many hospitals—people are still expected to lay quietly in bed (preferably with an epidural), give birth on their backs with their feet in stirrups, and have things done to their vagina without consent.[83] And the Twilight Sleep movement and campaign to discredit midwives have resulted in a home birth rate in the U.S. of only 1%.[76]

Once my eyes were opened to the history of how midwifery and home birth had been systematically eliminated in the U.S., I felt like I'd been duped. This whole time—my whole childhood, adolescence, and young adult life—I'd been led to believe that it was normal and safest to find an obstetrician to attend the birth of your baby, and that birth should take place in a hospital. That was *just what you did* when you got pregnant! I'd had no idea that medical professionals of the first half of the 1900s had worked so hard to either eliminate midwifery or tightly regulate it for sexist, racist, and financial reasons, and to ensure that women only gave birth in hospitals. The worst part is, we all bought into it! We believed the lie! We either forgot about midwives entirely (like many young people I know, who don't know what a midwife is), or we view midwives as an "inferior" choice or home birth as "unsafe." One hundred years later, nobody stops to think about how all this came about!

I knew that in order to get the birth preferences I'd outlined, I absolutely had to find a midwife who could attend me in a home birth. But I had two problems—first, I had to convince Dan that home birth with a midwife was the right choice for our family. Second, how would I find a midwife, now that they were so scarce?

Convincing Dan was actually pretty easy. Although he was initially reluctant to consider the idea of a home birth, I did two things. First, I made him sit down with me and watch videos of several home births with midwives. Then, a few weeks later, I emailed him my carefully researched table of the benefits and risks of home birth vs. hospital birth, highlighting the research statistics on populations like me (low-risk people who have already had a successful vaginal birth before).

He said, "Okay, then."

Finding a midwife was much harder.

At first, when I started looking for a midwife, I had trouble figuring out if home birth was legal or not. I spent several hours on the Internet, searching, "Is home birth legal in my state?" I pored over message boards and blog articles, and finally uncovered that it was legal for *me* to give birth wherever I wanted. I could go to the local restaurant and give birth in a bathroom stall if I wanted to! However, thanks to that propaganda campaign from the early 1900s, there were very few midwives left in my state. There were a few nurse-midwives in my region, but only one attended home births, and she wasn't available during my due date. And about 40 years earlier, my state had stopped issuing permits to direct-entry midwives. There were a few direct-entry midwives who practiced "underground," but they could be charged with a misdemeanor if the state decided to prosecute them.

Before I go any further, let me clarify some of the different types of midwives in the U.S. A direct-entry midwife is someone who goes straight into studying midwifery, without going through nursing school beforehand. Direct-entry midwifery is quite common around the world. In the U.S., the direct-entry Certified Professional Midwife (CPM) credential was inaugurated in 1994. About half of all CPMs graduate from an accredited midwifery education program, and the other half learn the profession through a formal apprenticeship. Regardless of which educational path they take, all CPMs must learn the same content and take the same national certification examination.[74, 91]

The most common type of midwife in the U.S. is a Certified Nurse-Midwife (CNM)—a midwife who goes through nursing school first, and then completes an academic graduate program in nurse-midwifery. CNMs graduate with Master's degrees, and are qualified to provide not only labor and delivery care, but also well-woman care throughout the course of a woman's lifespan.[74, 91]

In the U.S., CNMs work primarily in hospital settings, while CPMs work only in community settings—in freestanding birth centers and at home births. Yet in almost every other part of the world, direct-entry midwives work in both hospital and community settings. Interestingly, the U.S. is the only country with such a split system of professional midwifery.[74]

After reviewing all my options, I was faced with a dilemma: I could have a home birth, but it would have to be with an underground CPM, if I could find one. Was that worth the risk? Legally, it wasn't a risk for me, but it would be for my midwife. I was worried. Did I want to do something that had even a hint of illegality about it? However, my fear of repeating a traumatic hospital birth was greater than my fear of hiring an underground midwife. So I decided to keep exploring the option.

I was still seeing my obstetrician from my former birth, the same one who helped me have a vaginal birth by giving me plenty of time to push. At one of my early prenatal visits, I tentatively brought up the fact that I was considering a home birth this time around. I then froze, afraid of what she might say.

She smiled, and said something like, "You know, the American Congress of Obstetricians and Gynecologists wants me to tell you that home birth is not safe, but actually, you're a really good candidate for a home birth."[92]

She then promised to back me up and be my physician if, for some reason, I needed to transfer from home to the hospital.

Next, I found someone who was willing to secretly share the contact info of an underground midwife. Feeling shy and a bit reluctant, I dialed the number. Karen Brown, a CPM, answered the phone. After I explained why I was calling, she asked me to share my first birth story. I could tell she'd heard similar stories from distressed moms many times before, yet with her, I felt heard. I told her what I wanted for this birth, and she reassured me that everything on my list was something she did at nearly every birth.

We invited Karen to come to our home so that Dan could meet her and we could do a formal interview. We had a long list of questions to ask: What would she do in the event of an emergency? What medical supplies and equipment did she bring to the birth? What if the baby needed to be resuscitated? How did she handle transfers to the hospital? How many years of experience did she have? How many of her clients ended up needing Cesareans in the hospital? How many births had she attended? Who would she bring with her to be an assistant at the birth? How would she handle a postpartum hemorrhage? And so on.

Karen answered the questions with ease and professionalism, and Dan and I both felt an instant rapport with her. After Karen left and we closed the front door behind her, Dan turned to me and said, "Let's hire her."

However, before we took that step, I needed to do one last thing to safeguard myself. Karen had given me a reference list, with names and contact info of several past clients and nurse-midwives she had trained under. I called all of them, and the info they gave me was reassuring. According to the parents and legally practicing nurse-midwives I spoke with, Karen was a competent, professional, and safe practitioner. She had an excellent reputation in the community. We would be in good hands if we hired her.

I dialed her again. "Karen?" I said. "We would love to hire you to be our midwife, if you would have us."

"Of course!" she answered.

We were off! We began meeting with Karen for prenatal visits, in which she came to our home. Unlike my 5- or 10-minute appointments with my OB, each appointment with Karen was about an hour long. Not only did she do all the same health checks and tests that my OB did, but she spent a lot of time talking with me about improving my nutritional status, how to cope with my migraines (just like last time, my migraines worsened during pregnancy), and how I would integrate a second child into my life. Clara often cuddled with me on the couch during my appointments, and Karen would enlist her "help" to measure my abdomen and listen to the baby's heart rate. What was even more fun was how much time we spent talking and preparing for the birth! At each appointment, Karen gave me a new childbirth book to read or a video to watch. She also told me that even though this was my second go-around, that she required a childbirth class, and she handed me a list of recommended classes.

The class that Dan and I took ended up being amazing—so much better than that hospital class I'd taken during my first pregnancy. My sister Shannon, who was finishing up residency, mentioned that her clients who used self-hypnosis seemed to have really smooth, comfortable labors. I knew I couldn't have an epidural this time since they aren't used in home births, so I wanted to learn as many comfort measure strategies as possible! I looked into classes on self-hypnosis for childbirth. I found out that there were two popular curricula in the U.S.—one was called Hypnobirthing®, and another was called Hypnobabies®. There was a Hypnobabies® Instructor located near me, so I signed us up for the next class.

In our Hypnobabies® class, we spent a lot of time learning self-hypnosis techniques, and a big part of that training included addressing our fears about birth. One way we lowered fear was through changing the language we used about birth. Instead of saying "delivery," which implies that the doctor does all the work, we said that we are "giving birth." Instead of "contractions," which has connotations of pain, we called them "pressure waves." Instead of "labor," which sounds really hard, we called it our "birthing time." I began to spend time prepping and training my body *and* mind for being able to deeply relax during my birthing time.

All those people who say you can't prepare for something so unpredictable? They're wrong. The beauty of a really good childbirth class is that it can prepare you *to cope with the unpredictable nature* of birth. I practiced my self-hypnosis skills over and over until I could go into a deeply relaxed state with literally the drop of a finger (this is called the "finger-drop" technique in Hypnobabies®). There's something so wonderful about that state of mind—I always felt so relaxed, yet alert, and almost euphoric afterwards. We did a birthing rehearsal in our last class, and I felt amazing. I loved pretending like I was giving birth! I couldn't wait for the real thing!

And then, a few months before I was due with my second, Shannon, my own sister, gave birth to her first child. She had a long, exhausting (but perfectly healthy) pregnancy, working a total of 80 hours per week as a resident, capped off with a 30-hour-long call shift at the end of every week (yes—working 30 hours in a row!).

Shannon was determined to have an unmedicated birth. She and her husband studied the Bradley® method, which focuses on preparing the husband to be the labor coach. However, their plans were sidetracked by the fact that two weeks past her due date, labor still hadn't started yet. Shannon had days and days of prodromal labor, where she'd have contractions that wouldn't get into a regular pattern, and would eventually fizzle out. At 42 weeks and 0 days, she checked into the university hospital for a medical labor induction—the same hospital where I had given birth to Clara.

Being a resident doctor and an insider in the hospital gave Shannon a few advantages that most people don't have. Not only did she bring a doula with her, but she hand-picked the OB resident in charge of her care. Shannon had already educated herself on the evidence ahead of time, she knew exactly what she wanted, and she was prepared to fight for what she wanted if she had to. She'd even made several back-up birth plans in the event of an induction or Cesarean!

Shannon ended up refusing as many interventions as possible with an induction. She kept saying, "No, thank you," "No, thank you," "No, thank you" every time the nurses tried to tell her she needed various interventions, such as IV fluids. She also took breaks off the fetal monitor to go to the bathroom, and she spent time laboring in the hospital shower.

Shannon was induced with misoprostol, also known as Cytotec®, a drug that is highly effective at inducing labor, but has the potential side effect of creating particularly intense, frequent contractions. Shannon and her husband used every comfort measure skill they'd practiced, and made it through 12 hours of hard, Cytotec-induced labor without any pain medication. When her daughter was born, Shannon felt an overwhelming sense of pride and exhilaration. She told me that she felt empowered because she had stood up for herself and gave birth the way she wanted.

The nurse assigned to Shannon was kind and respectful. But Shannon, content with how everything had turned out, had no idea what was going on outside her room while she was in labor. Months later, she found out from another resident that other nurses had been gossiping about her and *mocking* her at the nurses' station. The nurses complained that she'd waited until 42 weeks to labor, and that she shouldn't have attempted unmedicated birth.

The specific words that they used? Shannon was "stupid," and she would have a "huge baby."

Shannon had a beautiful birth, and her daughter only weighed 7 pounds.

I was expecting a holiday baby this time, in December 2011. Nobody except our closest family knew we were planning a home birth. I was afraid of being judged or shamed for my choice. So, we kept our birth plans under wraps.

A few days after my due date, I woke up at 6 a.m. with a pressure wave. I shook Dan awake. "Dan, wake up! This is it!" I was excited and joyful—I couldn't wait to meet my baby! Dan called Karen, and she came over right away.

For the rest of the day, I relaxed, got in and out of the tub, had snacks and meals (we ate fresh cinnamon rolls!), and drank iced tea and lemonade. Briana, our babysitter, got Clara out of the house for a while—they baked cookies and delivered them to a nearby fire station. Karen monitored my baby's heart rate with a handheld Doppler device. At one point, I started to get tired, and Karen encouraged me to take a nap. I had trained my body to use self-hypnosis so well (those daily self-hypnosis practice sessions during pregnancy paid off!), I was able to sleep soundly through an hour of pressure waves!

When I woke up from my nap at around 4 p.m., things started happening faster. I got in the tub, and the intensity of the waves picked up, but I was feeling so, so happy! And get this—the waves actually were not painful! My use of the self-hypnosis was successful—all I felt was a sensation of pressure during the waves. In between each wave, I smiled, took a sip of water, and laughed and joked with Dan.

Then things got more intense. I was in the soft, inflatable tub on my knees, draping my upper body over the edge. Dan and I had been in the room by ourselves—Karen came in every 15 minutes or so to check on me and baby, but for the most part she was giving us privacy, because she said that would help labor progress. Dan was doing an amazing job being my support person, reading me Hypnobabies® scripts out loud and helping me stay calm and in self-hypnosis.

All of a sudden, my lower body spontaneously started pushing the baby out, and for the first time in 11 hours of labor, I felt pain.

"I need Karen!" I called out to Dan, suddenly feeling desperate and out of control.

Karen and her assistant were just outside the door, and as soon as she heard me call, she immediately came to my side. I wasn't even intentionally trying to push; it felt like my body was throwing the baby out. Kind of like that heaving sensation of throwing up, but from your bottom, if that makes sense. I found out later that this is called the fetal ejection reflex, and it happens most often with truly undisturbed birth (when you feel completely private and safe).[93]

Within 15 minutes of my body starting to push on its own, my baby was being born in the warm water!

Karen told me, firmly, "Rebecca, reach down and grab your baby!"

I gasped. "I can't do it!"

And she said, "Yes, you can, just reach down and grab your baby!"

I reached down and felt a baby in between my legs. I lifted him up to my chest and twirled around in the water. All of a sudden, there was this huge, pink baby lying on top of me.

"I did it! I did it!" I cried.

We hadn't known what the sex would be.

It was a boy.

Henry was perfectly calm and content, not crying, simply lying on my chest—his eyes gazing into mine. His Apgar scores were 10 and 10—as healthy as you can get. Our son had just entered the world, and I'd never had so much as one vaginal exam.

My sister-in-law brought Clara into the room, and Clara looked on with wide eyes at her mommy and baby brother in the tub. A little while later, Henry and I moved to the bed and we cuddled together as a family—Dan, myself, Clara, and Henry. I did skin-to-skin with Henry and nursed him, and when I got up to go to the bathroom, Dan got to do his skin-to-skin time with our new son—something he was never able to do with Clara.

After about an hour of bonding time, Karen and her assistant completed the newborn exam together. My family and birth attendants gathered around the bed to watch—laughing, oohing, and ahhing at how cute he was. My midwife asked if we had any guesses as to how much the new family member weighed. I guessed 8 pounds. Dan's brother Greg, who had just arrived at our house to see the baby, had the highest guess at 8 pounds 10 ounces.

Remember—my first baby was 6.5 pounds, and it took me three full hours, plus vacuum assistance, to push her out. Well, Henry was a chunk—and I had pushed him out in 15 minutes flat.

I heard his weight called out: "9 pounds, 2 ounces, 22 inches long."

I was stunned.

I thought, "I did that?? My body did that?? If I can do that, I can do anything!"

Throughout the rest of the evening, Karen spent several hours with me and Henry, making sure everything was normal, keeping an eye on our breastfeeding, and helping me get through those first hours of recovery.

During one trip to the bathroom, as Karen helped me walk, I remember pausing and asking her, "When do we give him his first bath?"

She said, "Rebecca, he's your baby. You can give him a bath whenever you want!"

I thought, "You're right. He *is* my baby!"

Not discounting all the wonderful clinical care Karen provided, the best gift she ever gave me was this—the knowledge and empowerment that *I* was the mother of this baby. Nobody was going to take my baby away and give him a bath without asking me first. I was his mother. I was going to be parenting him and making a whole bunch of decisions for him in his first years of life. The decision of when to give him his first bath was totally up to me, and no one else.

Although this realization was delightful and heartwarming, I couldn't help but immediately think back to Clara's birth and the first three hours of her life, when she lay alone and naked in an isolette in the nursery, with nobody even keeping an eye on her.

To this day, all of my children share the love language of touch. They love to cuddle, give back rubs, receive back rubs, and just be close to us physically. How traumatic must it have been for Clara to lie there for her first 3 hours on earth, by herself, with no one touching her or picking her up, except for when they did clinical procedures? What kind of trauma was it for me, to not be allowed to hold her?

The truth is, I can never get those hours back. I can do everything I can to make it up to my daughter today, by loving her and cuddling her, but I can *never* get those first hours back.

For the rest of my life, I will regret that we were separated from each other during those crucial hours after birth.

The difference between the two types of care I had received was stark. At Clara's birth, I'd been coerced into unnecessary interventions, starved, restricted from moving or going to the bathroom, and then finally separated unnecessarily from the baby who had lived inside my body for nine months beforehand.

With Henry, I'd been supported and cared for, given options, kept comforted and safe, given privacy when needed, and encouraged to stay skin-to-skin with a baby who was recognized as fully mine.

Although I had set out to get a birth that I viewed as "evidence based," I'd ended up with so much more. I ended up with the realization that I could do anything, that I was powerful as a human being and a mother, and that more people deserved this type of empowering care—in every birth setting, with every type of birth, and with every type of provider.

As I nursed my new baby, and marveled at his chunky cheeks and full head of hair, I realized that I had just had a ground-shaking reorganization of my life's work. Originally, I had just wanted to get evidence based care for this birth. That was my only goal. Now I had a new goal. I knew I would—and could—do anything to help as many people as possible get better care. To help other people avoid that cookie-cutter American experience of childbirth that leaves so many people feeling broken and scarred, and instead help people find the kind of birth that leaves them feeling empowered and strong.

I looked down at baby Henry, and glanced at my now-three-year-old Clara, who was cuddling next to my side. I had a new mission. By the time both my babies were grown up and having babies of their own, they wouldn't have to fight to get evidence based care. For them, evidence based care would be a given.

Chapter Four

TAKE-OFF

BEFORE HENRY'S BIRTH, I was looking forward to giving birth at home, but afraid and ashamed to tell anyone about my choices. Now, I had an incredible amount of energy (quite unusual for someone who is freshly postpartum), my migraines were completely gone, and I wanted to tell my birth story to anyone who would listen!

At four weeks postpartum, I took Henry with me to campus and shared photos from his birth with my former nursing students from the fall semester, who were now in their spring obstetrical rotation. The students were enthralled by my home birth and asked me countless questions.

"How much does a home birth cost?"

"What was the pain like?'

"What would you recommend I do, so that I can get evidence based care when I start a family?

"How do you find a midwife?"

After my guest lecture was over, I was approached by several students who were distraught by what they'd been seeing in labor and delivery—patients being openly ridiculed for their birth plan; patients being shamed for their body weight during labor; healthy patients being pressured into procedures they didn't want or need.

The students asked me, "What should we do when we see care that's not evidence based?"

I didn't know what to say, but I encouraged them to educate themselves as much as possible about evidence based care, to advocate for their patients, and to choose the best health care team possible for their own births in the future.

Then, while still on maternity leave, I got an email from an attending physician in the family medicine department at my university. She wanted me to come speak with their family medicine residents about my two very different birth experiences and about midwifery care. I accepted the invitation immediately.

As I prepared for my talk with these residents, I wondered what might be most helpful for them. So, I emailed the attending physician and asked what she thought.

She responded, "If you have any evidence you can share with us, we're always looking for evidence on which we can base our practice."

"Ah ha," I thought. "*That* I can help with."

By this point, I had collected a treasure trove of research articles about the evidence on different childbirth practices. I thought of four non-evidence based practices that the residents would benefit from learning about, and that were still a problem at this hospital:

- Forbidding eating and drinking
- Requiring confinement to bed during labor
- Requiring IV fluids
- Requiring continuous electronic fetal monitoring

I took the evidence I'd gathered on these topics and created a one-page handout for each topic. I printed enough copies for all the residents and headed off to give my talk.

Henry slept in my baby-wearing wrap while I shared my two birth experiences with the residents. First, using the projector, I showed photos from my first birth, including photos of Clara lying by herself in the isolette in the nursery. Next, I showed photos from my second birth, in which I received care from a midwife. The residents listened attentively, asked questions, and lamented their current situation. They told me that they wanted to improve practices at their hospital, but felt like their hands were tied by the obstetricians and nurses, who did not support the midwifery model of care, much less the family medicine model of care (a holistic care model that has similarities to the midwifery model). The residents really perked up when I handed out the evidence I'd compiled. They each took their copies, and were reading them over, when the attending physician said, "These are excellent. Do you have any handouts about the evidence on other topics?"

"Hmm," I thought. "If they found these handouts helpful, maybe other people would!"

I went home and was happily telling Dan about my talk with the residents when a solution popped into my head. Out of nowhere, I blurted out, "Dan . . . I'm starting a blog!"

Starting a blog isn't all that unusual these days, but I was already pretty busy to be taking this on. I was going back to work in a few weeks, and I was a full-time working parent in an intense tenure-track faculty position, while Dan worked full-time as an accountant for a technology firm. A lot of pressure to get grant funding came along with my job—thankfully, so far, I'd been successful. The morning I was in labor with Henry, I'd checked my email (remember, I had a mostly painless labor!) and found out I would be awarded a $356,000 grant from the National Institutes of Health to complete a 3-year training program and conduct a randomized trial on cognitive behavioral therapy for patients with heart disease! I knew that as soon as the grant money hit the university bank account, I would be starting that new clinical trial. And now we had a 3-year old and a newborn. But I also knew, without a doubt, that starting a blog was something I absolutely *had* to do!

I opened a blank Word document on my computer and started brain-dumping potential blog titles. I Googled "evidence based maternity care," and didn't find any websites like the one I envisioned. Just like that, the phrase "Evidence Based Birth" popped into my head. It struck me as a catchy blog title, and maybe even potentially a movement! I purchased the domain name "EvidenceBasedBirth.com," checked out a book from the library called "Blogging for Dummies," and figured out how to create a free blog from scratch. And so it was that on March 30, 2012, I began posting the research findings I'd been collecting about childbirth.

I thought, "Maybe ten or twelve people will find these articles. If it helps just a few people, I'll be happy."

I waited until there were a few blog articles on the site before sharing it with anyone. A few weeks later, I sat at my desk at home, feeling nervous, and finally worked up the courage to "share" the link to my blog on my personal Facebook page. I was stunned and a little frightened when the Facebook post started getting attention right away! First my prenatal yoga instructor shared the link to my new blog. Then Karen, my midwife. Everyone seemed to be sharing my articles on Facebook. Within a few weeks, totally random bloggers, whom I'd never met, began writing blog articles about my articles—directing people to my website!

I realized I had discovered a huge problem in need of a solution. Consumers and so many professionals in the childbirth field were excited about evidence based care, but it wasn't truly available in many labor and delivery units, and people wanted to soak up anything they could read about it.

I started to brainstorm ways I could use my energy and excitement about evidence based practice to create change at my university's labor and delivery unit. Maybe I was still feeling empowered from my amazing birth with Henry. Or maybe I was just naïve. But for some reason, a little over a month after I started my blog, I emailed the nurse administrator who oversaw the university's labor and delivery unit and asked for a meeting to discuss some feedback I had about my birth experience, and to talk about what other women were telling me about their own experiences there.

One week passed, and I didn't receive a response. Two weeks—nothing. Discouraged, I told a few of my fellow nursing professors about how I wasn't getting any response. One of them had a good relationship with a different nurse administrator. She emailed that second nurse, and within hours, the second nurse emailed me back. It turned out that the first nurse administrator had gotten my email—she just didn't respond. We set up a meeting for mid-June.

A few weeks later, I sat in a white-walled office in the women and children's hospital. As everyone was settling into their chairs, I glanced out the window, overlooking the hospital's air conditioning units, then turned my eyes back to the three nurses sitting across from me at the table. I smiled, introduced myself, and explained why I'd asked for the meeting. I told them how I'd felt like I was limited in my choices when I gave birth there nearly four years ago, and now mothers from all over the region were coming to me, saying that they were still having the same problems. In preparation for this meeting, I'd done an informal survey of mothers and doulas in the area, gathering their "wish list" for the university labor and delivery department. The top three items on the wish list were

- Tubs for water immersion during labor
- Intermittent auscultation as an option instead of continuous electronic fetal monitoring for everyone
- Permission to eat and drink during labor

The nursing administrators then proceeded to explain point by point why none of these requests were reasonable.

They said that they empathized with me, and they were sorry I felt that I hadn't had a good birth experience in their facility.

They told me, "We want women to have good experiences!"

They said, "We try to accommodate women's birth plans whenever possible."

They then gave the example of a woman who had recently requested to have five support people present during her labor—their policy was only to permit four support persons.

However, since the woman's relatives were well-behaved, they were willing to make an exception to the policy in her unique case, and they allowed the additional person to be present at the birth. It seemed like an odd example to me.

But otherwise, I was told, some things, like intermittent auscultation instead of electronic fetal monitoring, and providing tubs for water immersion, or permitting women to eat and drink during labor, were just not going to happen. Ever.

I was told the nurses can't be allowed to do intermittent auscultation "because they don't do it enough to be comfortable doing it." They also said they don't have enough nurses, and "it's easier to just put everyone on the monitor and watch the patients from the nursing station."

I left the meeting feeling totally deflated.

I had gone in excited and hopeful, thankful to have an opportunity to talk respectfully and face to face with decision-makers, with nurse colleagues. But it seemed to me, from watching body language and verbal cues, that one of the nurse administrators in particular (the one who never returned my email), was adamantly opposed to the requests I'd brought forward. And none of them seemed to have any interest in learning new research evidence on these topics. I had a gut feeling that these nurses had met with me out of politeness, since they were friends with the professor who connected us, but that they did not have any intention of changing anything.

As time passed, I struggled with understanding what was going on here. Why was it *so* difficult to change culture in one small nursing unit? And how is it that two or three people—a couple of administrators—can hold back everyone else from progress, limiting families' choices? And it wasn't just the clinicians in my hospital, either . . . I'd begun to understand that other hospitals across the country had similar problems.

"Why?" I asked myself. "Why are some people so resistant to change?"

This question tugged at my brain. So, as usual, I started looking at the research! Since I couldn't find anything published in medical journals about resistance to change in labor and delivery units, I turned to the research about change in general, much of which comes from the field of social psychology.

Social psychology seeks to understand why individuals act the way they do in certain social situations. Years after this meeting, as I continued to learn everything I could about social psychology, I discovered the Audible course, "Why You Are Who You Are: Investigations into Human Personality" by Dr. Mark Leary, a professor at Duke University.[94] In the very first chapter of his course, I learned from Dr. Leary that problematic behaviors, like a nurse's resistance to change, are personality problems.

Dr. Leary teaches that there are five key personality traits that exist in some degree, whether low or high, in all of us: extroversion, neuroticism, agreeableness, conscientiousness, and openness. While listening to his course, four of these qualities struck me as traits that could contribute to health care worker resistance to change. Don't worry, extroversion is *not* a trait that influences resistance to change, so whether you're an extrovert or introvert, I'm not going to complain about you! However, these are the four traits that can be problematic:

> **Neuroticism** refers to the degree to which people experience negative emotions like anxiety or sadness. If a health

care worker is *high in neuroticism*, they are probably heavily focused on avoiding risks, including avoiding anything that could be construed as a threatening situation. They may also overreact to normal stressors.

Agreeableness is the tendency to have a positive view toward other people. If a health care worker is *low in agreeableness*, they may be less trusting of a patient's decision, more inconsiderate or calloused about patients' feelings, more confrontational, and more prejudiced toward stigmatized groups, such as minorities.

Conscientiousness refers to how responsible and self-disciplined you are. Typically, conscientiousness is seen as a positive trait. However, health care workers who are *high in conscientiousness* (like many nurses I know) can also be hyper-focused on maintaining social norms and on making sure that policies and doctors' orders are carefully followed.

Openness means how receptive you are to new ideas. People who are high in openness show a kind of intellectual curiosity that makes them excited to learn about new evidence or new ways of doing things. But health care workers who are *low in openness* don't like to try new things. They are dogmatic, conventional, set in their ways, and quite certain that *their* beliefs are correct—not yours.

After taking Dr. Leary's course, everything clicked for me, especially the concept of openness. I knew that I must be high in openness—I'm incredibly curious and excited about improving health care practices. But some of these people I was bumping up to in labor and delivery seemed to be low in openness, hyper-focused on maintaining social norms, and anxious at every turn about the fear of "something going wrong." Unfortunately, people with these types of personality traits—especially if they're in positions of power—can hold others back from making any sort of culture change.

But let's back up a minute—why would we need leaders to change *culture* in order to make change? Why is the culture of the labor and delivery unit so important, and what does that have to do with evidence based care?

Well, culture is defined as the subtle, taken-for-granted, but incredibly powerful context that shapes our lives, workplaces, and organizations. The culture of a hospital is not the values that they print on a poster. Instead, it's the default beliefs, group norms, and behaviors, usually never scrutinized or examined, that drive the daily behaviors and actions of hospital staff. In other words, it's "the way we do things around here."[95,96]

Here are some examples of key elements of "the way we do things around here" that might be hostile to patient autonomy or evidence based options in childbirth:[3]

> **Physical artifacts:** Reliance upon continuous electronic fetal monitoring equipment for every single patient, outdated triage rooms with no privacy, the hospital bed as the focus of the room (no props or tubs or furniture that might encourage clients to be upright and mobile), the ubiquitous use of stirrups for lithotomy (back-lying or semi-sitting) position during the pushing phase.
>
> **Language and jargon:** Saying the doctor will "deliver" your baby, using dehumanizing language ("I have to go do a vag exam on the induction in room 40"), and using authoritative language ("You're *not allowed* to eat during labor" or "We *can't let you* get out of bed.").

Stories, myths, and legends: Telling myths such as "eating and drinking is dangerous during labor," "standing up after your water has broken will cause the cord to prolapse," "vaginal birth after Cesarean is too risky and should not be attempted," and "if you go past your due date you have a 50% chance of stillbirth" (none of these are true!).

Behavioral norms: Nurses spend most of their time at the nurse's station (watching the central monitor rather than being in the room with the patient), nurses manage the second stage of labor and dictate how and when the mother pushes, the doctor comes in at the very last minute just for the birth of the baby.

Shared values and beliefs: Labor is something to be managed with as many interventions as possible—including but not limited to Pitocin®, intravenous fluids, and artificial rupture of membranes; epidurals are beneficial for pain control PLUS they benefit staff because they keep the patient quiet, in bed, and on the monitor; legal risks to the hospital should be managed at all costs, even if it means limiting a patient's choice or forbidding evidence based options such as intermittent auscultation.

Rituals: Asking the birthing person to put on a hospital gown when they are admitted, performing frequent vaginal exams, turning on the bright ceiling spotlights as the baby is being born, clamping the cord within 60 seconds, sending the baby to the newborn nursery for routine tests and exams instead of having these procedures done in the mother's room.

After reading these examples, you might get the feeling, like I did, that hospital culture is really, really powerful. I mean, it's an entire world with its own language, and customs, and beliefs. In retrospect, my attempt to meet with the administrators seemed feeble and kind of ridiculous. What chance does an ordinary person, like me, have against this force?

But, I reminded myself, the traffic to Evidence Based Birth had really taken off in the past few weeks. I wondered . . . maybe I could make an impact in a different way, or in a different place?

My mind was drawn to an important lesson I'd learned a while back from *Seven Habits of Highly Effective People*, by Dr. Stephen Covey.[97] Dr. Covey teaches that there are two circles we encounter in life—the Circle of Concern and the Circle of Influence.

The *Circle of Concern* includes all of the things we worry about—our family, our health, our job, our education, but also things that are completely out of our hands, like wars, famine, political events, and more. The *Circle of Influence* is much smaller, and it includes only those things we have direct or indirect influence over.

Covey's theory is that if we spend time worrying about things in our Circle of Concern, but that we have no Influence over, that this creates a negative energy that shrinks our Circle of Influence.

But if we focus on what we can actually do inside our Circle of Influence, and put all our energy toward that, over time, our Circle of Influence expands to include more items in the Circle of Concern.

I realized that my university hospital was in my Circle of Concern, but definitely *not* in my Circle of Influence.

I decided to try to ignore what was going on there, and instead devote myself, as much as possible, to my Circle of Influence. For the time being, that meant focusing all my spare time on writing about evidence based care and getting it into the hands of families and professionals in other communities. Because if I did that—if I went straight to other families, maybe they could use their voices, in combination with mine, to demand evidence based care and create change.

Could this strategy work? I wasn't sure. But there wasn't anything else I could do, and doing nothing wasn't an option. And so, I dove head first into writing. During the weekdays, I worked at my faculty job. But every weekend when my kids were napping, every Friday night when Clara was watching a movie, and for an hour or two after the kids' bedtime every single weeknight, I was writing. Searching for research, reading research, and writing. It felt like I was driven by something higher than me. The future health of my children depended on my ability to fix the maternity care system before they had children of their own.

At least, I thought that was who I was writing for. But very quickly I would realize that my blog readers, all of whom were wholly unrelated to me, also depended upon the work I was doing.

Chapter Five

POWER

THE FIRST PRIVATE MESSAGE I received about Evidence Based Birth was from someone named Sarah Wylie (Sarah Wylie is her first name, not her first and last names). A few weeks after my meeting with the nurse administrators at my hospital, Sarah Wylie's message popped up in my inbox. She introduced herself as a fellow Hypnobabies® mom who worked at my university and therefore had to give birth there.

Sarah Wylie had hired a doula, and in one of their prenatal conversations, the doula dropped a hint that Sarah Wylie's obstetrician probably wouldn't be present at the birth.

"What do you mean?" she asked.

"Well," the doula said cautiously, "the doctors in that practice rotate call. Your doctor might be supportive of your birth plan, but the others might not be."

"Does that really matter?" Sarah Wylie asked. "I mean, the doctor only comes in at the very end, right? How much influence can they have over whether or not I'm allowed to get everything on my birth plan?"

"A lot," the doula said.

Concerned, Sarah Wylie asked for help in switching care providers. She found out that there was a family medicine residency program at the same hospital, in which all the residents practiced continuity of care. Some family medicine residents enjoyed working with doulas and patients who had unmedicated births. So, Sarah Wylie switched from an attending obstetrician (with a lot of power) to a family medicine resident (with significantly less power). She learned pretty quickly that the trade-off was worth it. At her first appointment with the resident, Sarah Wylie felt an instant connection. It was a patient-provider match made in heaven!

Sarah Wylie told me she loved the new Evidence Based Birth blog. She was about to give birth to her first child, a boy, and she wanted tips on how to get the hospital staff to accept her birth plan. She had recently found out about intermittent auscultation, and she really wanted that to be part of her care. She also wanted to refuse an IV or saline lock (unless it became medically necessary). In short, she wanted two things the university hospital never did.

Sarah Wylie told me that she thought that as long as she stuck to her ground, refused the IV, and refused to be put on the electronic fetal monitor, that there was nothing the hospital staff could do. She hoped these things wouldn't be too big a deal. Sarah Wylie had heard that the nurses at the hospital didn't know how to do intermittent auscultation, but her resident had been trained in this by midwives at another hospital, so the resident could do it instead.

By the time she initially reached out to me, Sarah Wylie was already a few days past her due date. There wasn't much time left to prepare the hospital for her new requests. But she decided to go for it anyway. What's the worst that could happen?

Several days passed, and I didn't hear from Sarah Wylie. Then, I finally got word from her: She'd had her baby, Otis, and she'd managed to have a completely unmedicated, low-intervention birth in the hospital! Both she and her baby were healthy.

But, that's not the full story.

Sarah Wylie went a little over a week past her due date. She went into labor spontaneously, and called the resident to give her a heads-up. Sarah Wylie labored at home all day with her husband. The "pressure waves" were easy for her to handle. When it came time for her to drive to the hospital, she stayed deeply in self-hypnosis, keeping her noise-canceling headphones on, and swaying and moaning with the pressure waves.

It was 10 p.m. when Sarah Wylie walked into the hospital. She was in active labor and needing a lot of support—her doula and husband Griffin stayed by her side. The pressure waves were coming every two to five minutes. She was 5 centimeters dilated, and the baby's heart rate was normal. So far, she was having a picture-perfect labor.

That's when things started to get complicated.

While Sarah Wylie checked into triage, her nurse looked at the birth plan and called the attending OB immediately, even though Sarah Wylie wasn't a patient of the OB department—she was technically a patient of the family medicine department. The next thing Sarah Wylie knew, an attending OB stood beside her stretcher, expressing deep concern that Sarah Wylie had declined the continuous electronic fetal monitor. Sarah Wylie explained that she wasn't declining monitoring all together—she wanted intermittent auscultation, instead.

The attending OB had never heard of it.

She said, "That's not monitoring. I need a strip. I can't do my job without a strip." (A strip is the computer read-out of the electronic monitor recording).

The OB kept talking, even when Sarah Wylie was moaning and in the middle of intense, frequent contractions. Sarah Wylie tried her best to stay focused.

She remembers the OB saying things like,

"You're placing your baby at risk," and

"Your baby could have a low pH," and

"Your baby could have brain damage," and

"Your baby could have fetal demise."

None of this was true, but Sarah Wylie knew her facts.

She just looked at the OB and calmly said, "No, thank you."

The attending OB marched right back out the door, and the next thing Sarah Wylie knew, they had refused to admit her to a labor and delivery room. Sarah Wylie remained stuck in triage on a stretcher.

The family medicine resident remained close to Sarah Wylie, encouraging her through the pressure waves, and monitoring the baby every 15 minutes with the Doppler.

Eventually the attending family medicine physician showed up as well. She tried to explain the safety of intermittent auscultation to the OB. By now, it was the middle of the night. The hospital risk management attorney and the chair of obstetrics were called (probably woken up at home from their sleep). Sarah Wylie doesn't know what was said in these conversations, but what we do know is that both the family medicine attending physician and the on-call attending obstetrician wrote very long handwritten notes about how they had informed the patient of the many "dangerous" risks of declining the electronic fetal monitor.

Finally, at around 12:30 a.m., more than two hours after she'd walked into the hospital in active labor, Sarah Wylie was allowed to be admitted into a real hospital room. At 3:19 a.m., after 1 hour and 19 minutes of pushing, Sarah Wylie gave birth to a healthy baby boy.

It's hard to express how disappointed and frustrated I was upon hearing how Sarah Wylie and her husband were treated. It was like re-living Clara's birth all over again—the pressure, the coercion, the inability to see each patient as an individual— the unfamiliarity with evidence based care. I was ashamed and upset that the staff were continuing to limit women's options during childbirth—that they didn't even know what the evidence said about intermittent auscultation vs. electronic fetal monitoring—evidence that had been confirmed repeatedly more than twenty years ago! The meeting I'd had with the nurse administrators had all been for nothing. Nothing was going to change.

But Sarah Wylie wasn't the only one who suffered for requesting evidence based care. The resident who cared for her was professionally retaliated against by the physicians and nurses. Why? She was viewed as a "troublemaker" for supporting Sarah Wylie's wishes.

Right now, you might be shaking your head. "What? What do you mean by retaliation? How is that even possible?"

There are a variety of ways that hospital administrators and nursing staff can exert their power over a physician, ranging from excluding them socially, to writing incident reports, to undermining them in front of patients, to sabotaging their quality improvement projects, to ridiculing them in meetings, to holding disciplinary hearings. However, one of the harshest punishments a hospital can inflict on a provider is a threat to deny, suspend, or revoke hospital privileges.

Before I define hospital privileges, let me back up and paint a picture for you. Imagine your life's dream was to become a doctor. You went to college and focused your studies on pre-med—enduring organic chemistry, physiology, and a host of other difficult science and math classes. You graduate with $26,900 in debt, or up to an average of $32,600 in debt if you went to a private university (although some people garner much more debt than that!)[98]

You bite your nails worrying about whether or not you can get into medical school. Good news! You made it in! You now spend the next four years of your life studying non-stop in the actual medical school program—with two of those years spent in both the classroom and clinical setting. Finally, you graduate! You now are likely to have an average of $197,000 in debt at graduation—$189,000 if you've gone to public universities, and $209,000+ if you've gone to private universities.[99] But you're done, right?

Oops, we forgot about residency! You are passionate about obstetrics, so after you pass your initial board exams and become an MD or DO, you apply/interview (another nail biter to find out if you got in or not!) and are matched with a program where you will spend the next four years as an obstetrics and gynecology resident, working 80 hours per week, and making an average of $13.70 per hour.[100] During this time span, you pass more board exams. Finally, you graduate from residency. By the way, you've just been hired into an obstetric practice! Congratulations—you can start paying off your debt!

In order to begin practicing in a hospital, you must first apply for credentials there.[101] After an extensive application process, the hospital approves your credentials. (Phew!) Next, your credentials will be reviewed by a governing medical board at the hospital. This board will decide to grant or deny you hospital privileges. Gaining hospital privileges is essential, because not only can you not practice in a hospital if you don't have privileges, but most health insurance plans will not allow their patients to see you unless you have privileges. Also, if your application is denied, it's possible that every other hospital in town will hear about it, and they might decide to deny you, too.

Once you have privileges at a hospital, you can begin to practice medicine there. However, if you're ever labeled a "disruptive physician"[102,103] (a vague term that can be used to target anyone who is not liked by administrators or peers, or who doesn't practice the way everybody else practices), or if you run across any other trouble, you may be called to a hospital-run disciplinary hearing. At that hearing, you have the right to be present and represent yourself. However, if you lose your case, the hospital could decide to suspend or revoke your privileges. Afterward, the hospital will likely report this event to a national database,[104] creating a red flag on your record.[105] It will be very difficult to get privileges at another hospital, and it's also going to be difficult to get insurance plans to reimburse you for patient care.[106,107]

If a care provider is concerned that they are being labeled as disruptive, there are several actions that they can take.[108] First, if there is even a hint that a colleague, patient, or administrator thinks that the provider's behavior is "disruptive," this situation should not be taken lightly. The care provider should not admit inappropriate conduct, and should seek legal counsel, so that the situation can be formally and immediately addressed. It's also important that the physician know the agenda of any meetings on the topic of their "disruptive conduct," as well as who is going to attend. They should demand that any accusation be confirmed from the source in writing, and their response should also be in writing. If the complaint is resolved, the resolution should be documented, and a copy provided to the physician and added to any relevant files kept on the physician.

Even though a care provider can seek legal help and take action to address accusations of being disruptive, you can imagine how stressful and anxiety-producing it might be for a care provider to be threatened with loss or suspension of privileges. Do you see how this system could be used to wield power over physicians who are seen as troublemakers for advocating for childbirth practices that aren't "routine" or "standard?" in your medical community? Maybe even evidence based, but locally disliked practices, such as intermittent auscultation, or even simple things like letting your client labor without an IV?

Say you were a doctor and had to choose between supporting your client's request for intermittent auscultation (and facing a hospital hearing about the future of your privileges) or sticking with the social norms and requiring electronic fetal monitoring (and avoiding any trouble with colleagues and administrators). Which would you choose?

This is not just a theoretical choice. I have communicated with physicians and midwives from all over the U.S. who have run into this problem: they want to protect their patient's right to make decisions about the birth of their baby, particularly evidence based decisions that are in line with the midwifery model of care. But if the provider does so, in some hospitals (although not all), this decision can come at a cost. And it's not just physicians, but also midwives who are at the mercy of this system.

A few years after Sarah Wylie and her resident experienced the fallout from requesting intermittent auscultation, Michelle, a certified nurse-midwife located in another state, was brought on board at a major regional medical center because they wanted to boost their delivery numbers—they were losing market share to hospitals that offered midwifery care. In that first year, Michelle recruited another CNM to practice with her, and their client base grew 220%.

After 16 months, however, hospital management closed down the labor and delivery unit, telling Michelle and her colleague that they would be moved to another hospital in the region. Sadly, the new hospital did not have any other midwives on staff, and had a reputation for being openly hostile to midwifery care. Michelle's colleague put in her notice before they moved to the new hospital, but Michelle decided to stick it out because she refused to abandon the many families who had already chosen her to attend their births.

In the two months that Michelle worked at the new hospital, she was "written up" for a variety of evidence based practices or for silly, non-medical reasons. In hospitals, writing someone up is typically done by nurses. It involves submitting a formal report or complaint to the higher-ups, and is usually done when a nurse witnesses serious breaches in ethics or safety. But write-ups can also occur simply because a nurse is upset or irritated by another nurse's or provider's practice decisions.

Michelle was written up by nurses for walking outside on campus for 15 minutes with an expectant couple, despite having okayed it with the nurse caring for the patient. She was written up for catching a baby with one glove on when the baby came too fast (this happens all the time to obstetric providers). She was written up for massaging a woman's lower back during labor without gloves, despite there being no bodily fluid exposure. She was written up for ordering intermittent auscultation on a patient who had reassuring and normal fetal heart tones. All of Michelle's clients, both mothers and babies, had healthy, normal birth outcomes. But that didn't matter.

The hospital held a hearing about Michelle. She was not allowed to attend the hearing to represent herself, nor was she told what the hearing was about. All she received was this vague communication: "There are several concerns that have been brought to the attention of the obstetrics department."

At the hearing, the chief medical officer of the hospital suspended Michelle's privileges.

Afterward, she was given the option of quitting or being fired. Michelle quit. She did not find out why her privileges were suspended until eight weeks after her forced resignation. She was told her care was "dangerous" and "outside community standards."

For the next year and a half, Michelle had to fight to get the suspension withdrawn. The process cost her $20,000 in legal fees, and during that time she was not eligible to get privileges at any other hospital or birthing center. Although she was successful in getting the suspension withdrawn, for the rest of her career, she has to disclose that her privileges were suspended temporarily, making it very difficult (and unlikely) for any other hospital to grant her privileges in the future.

Michelle switched to attending home births, which reduced her income by 90%. She obtained a part-time position in a family planning clinic to support the financial vagaries of a home birth practice. It took five months (rather than the typical 60–90 days) to get credentialed with one of the major health insurance providers in her state because of the hospital privilege suspension on her record. Another insurance carrier has still not approved her credentialing, and it's been seven months since she applied. This experience has made Michelle's ability to practice even in clinic settings precarious, likely for the remainder of her career.

Due to this series of events, Michelle suffered from significant clinical depression, suicidal thoughts, anxiety, and PTSD, for which she continues to receive therapy years later.

Now let's put yourself back into a patient's shoes. As a patient in the health care system, did you ever realize that your birth plan choices could be critiqued by a governing board at your hospital, and that this same board has the right to end your provider's career? Probably not. I have yet to meet a birthing family who realized this was a possibility, unless they themselves were physicians. For myself, this revelation was shocking. So much so that I couldn't stop thinking about it.

I would wake up in the middle of the night and my mind would race:

Why is it that even doctors and midwives don't have the power to create change in some hospitals?

If doctors can't create change, what hope do the rest of us have?

Why are their attempts to support patients in evidence based care blocked, and sometimes met with such hostility?

I knew that if I could just put my finger on the "why," I could maybe, eventually, help figure out a solution.

Then, finally, I uncovered a big part of the why.

I was sound asleep one night when I sprang awake at 4 a.m. with an idea: What if I look up research evidence about *systems of oppression*? Because that's really what this is, right? A system where people at the top of the power structure oppress people who are at the bottom? Maybe if I understand how this system functions, I can figure out how to create change!

I hopped out of bed, grabbed my laptop, sat down at the kitchen table, and spent the next three hours online, reading theories that describe how people with more societal power come to dominate people with less power. Through a Google search, I found a dissertation project published by a doctoral student, Teeomm Williams, from the University of Massachusetts Amherst. His paper was called "Understanding Internalized Oppression."[109] From reading Dr. Williams's work, I learned that there is an entire body of research on oppression, and most of it was done by researchers who studied systems of oppression related to racism and slavery. Dr. Williams's dissertation introduced me to a concept that would forever change how I viewed childbirth—Love's Pillars of Oppression Model, developed by Dr. Barbara Love.[110]

To help you understand what this Model of Oppression has to do with childbirth, let me show you something simple. I'm going to list a bunch of roles in our health care system in order, with the most powerful roles at the top, and the least powerful at the bottom:

> Hospital Administrator
> Hospital Lawyer
> Chief Obstetrician
> Obstetrician
> Family Physician who attends births
> Nurse Manager
> Midwife
> Resident
> Nurse
> Doula
> Student
> Birthing Person
> Partner
> Baby

This list depicts a typical hospital power hierarchy. But what are hierarchies? In the bestselling book, *Sapiens: A*

Brief History of Humankind, Dr. Yuval Noah Harari explains that hierarchies are when humans organize themselves into made-up groups.[111] The upper levels of the hierarchy have privileges and power, while the lower levels experience discrimination and oppression. It's eye-opening to realize, as Dr. Harari points out, that hierarchies are "all the product of human imagination." Yet, he reminds us that, "It is an iron rule of history that every imagined hierarchy disavows its fictional origins and claims to be natural and inevitable." I bring this up because I know some of you might say, "Well, so-and-so deserves to be at the top!"

Do they? Who gets to decide?

Today, I teach about the hospital power hierarchy to groups of families and professionals all across the United States. Whenever I do the power activity, I hand out signs labeled with the different roles and tell everyone to line up at the front of the room, in order from most powerful to least powerful. There may be slight differences in how the power structure is arranged, but nobody argues whether or not this power structure exists. Also, there's also a lot of consistency in who is typically labeled as having the "most power" at the top, and the "least power" at the bottom.

The people at the top of the power hierarchy are usually holding signs that say hospital lawyer, administrator, and chief obstetrician. When I ask them, "How does it feel to be at the top?" They usually reply, "Great!" or "Powerful!" although occasionally some of them say, "This feels like a heavy responsibility," or "I have a huge weight on my shoulders."

When I ask people at the bottom (usually the birthing person, partner, and baby) how it feels to be at the bottom, they say things like, "Small" or "Powerless" or "Nobody can hear me." Then I turn to people in the middle (nurses, midwives, and residents) and hand them toy swords. I ask them to start a battle. There's a lot of giggling as the nurses, midwives, and residents duke it out in the middle of the power chain.

But what upholds this system of oppression?

Imagine a building (this system of oppression) held up by two very strong pillars. These pillars, described by Dr. Love, hold up the system.

The first pillar that holds up the power hierarchy is called Oppressive Factors. These factors include

> Powerful individuals,
> Powerful institutions, and
> Culture

Powerful individuals in the childbirth care system have a lot of wealth, resources, privilege, and prejudice. When I think of powerful individuals, I think of hospital chief executives and vice presidents. Chief medical officers. Chief nursing officers. Chairs of obstetric departments. These people have a lot of power—a *lot*—and their leadership can determine the culture and practices of a hospital, for better or for worse. They can also be pretty arrogant, they are used to getting their way, and they are pretty far removed from the actual experiences that patients are having in their health care system.

Powerful institutions include laws, educational systems, hospitals, and professional trade associations. These institutions legitimize the power structure and build it into our social structure so we don't question it and can't challenge it. There were so many institutional Oppressive Factors happening in my state! For example, the medical schools and residency programs were graduating students who had never worked with midwives, leading to a workforce of physicians who were suspicious of midwives and their model of care. The American Congress of Obstetricians and Gynecologists and the state Hospital Association were actively lobbying against state bills that would legalize certified professional midwives—using their substantial power to crush bills about midwifery, sometimes before they could even get a hearing. Nurse-midwives were not being reimbursed fairly for their services by health insurance companies, so they could barely stay in business. There was a law stating that new nurse-midwives couldn't practice without finding a physician to "sign off" on their care, but physicians wouldn't agree to do so because they were suspicious of midwives. And on and on.

The third part of the Oppressive Factors pillar is culture. Our current culture in the United States—our values, rules, and norms—continues a 100-plus-year pattern of viewing midwives as "inferior" and telling parents that they should never question their doctors' decisions. Culture also means gaslighting someone who's had a traumatic birth by telling them they should "just be grateful you had a healthy baby." It means clinicians telling women that their babies are "too big" at the end of pregnancy, or nurses thinking that women with birth plans are "high maintenance." It means making (and believing) statements like "You're not allowed to eat during labor," or "Your pelvis isn't sufficient," or "If you don't have this induction, your baby's going to die."

So that's one pillar—the Oppressive Factors pillar.

The other pillar that holds up the power structure is called Internalized Oppression. Internalized Oppression is when people who are in the middle or bottom of the power structure—families, residents, midwives, doulas, nurses—accept the belief that they are inferior and worth less than people at the top. In my experience, most people don't realize that they have internalized these oppressive beliefs. But if you listen closely, you can hear it. Have you ever heard someone say: "I'm *just* a nurse," or "I'm *just* a mom," or "I'm *just* a doula?" This phrase is a classic symptom of Internalized Oppression!

But Internalized Oppression doesn't just create low self-confidence. It actually has well-known psychological and behavioral side effects! Psychological symptoms of Internalized Oppression include pain, powerlessness, suppressing your emotions, and feeling depressed, anxious, or traumatized. Behavioral symptoms include silence (not talking about what you're experiencing), feeling victimized, and showing constant deference to people who have more power than you. Also, the people who are oppressed know *a lot* about their oppressors. They know their likes, dislikes, and what might trigger an outburst or punishment. Meanwhile, the oppressors know very little about the people at the bottom of the hierarchy.

Another important symptom of Internalized Oppression is horizontal violence, which I demonstrate in the "power activity" I do with audiences when I ask nurses, midwives, and residents to carry out a sword fight. Although Styrofoam sword fights are silly, horizontal violence isn't. Horizontal violence is a form of lateral aggression between groups that have similarly low status. It's extremely common in female-dominated careers, such as midwifery and nursing, where people have a lot of responsibility but very little power.[112,113]

Have you ever heard the phrase, "Nurses eat their young?" That phrase refers to the fact that new nurses are sometimes abused by more experienced nurses. "Eating your young" is a form of horizontal violence—a cycle of trauma that persists from one generation to the next, and the next. I personally was a survivor of horizontal violence during my first year as a staff nurse—there were two charge nurses in particular who made me cry on a regular basis (not to mention threatened the safety of our patients by giving me impossible patient assignments)!

But it's not just nurses who sometimes eat their young. As Michelle told me in an email, "Oppression and professional assassination can come from all sides and within groups." Nurse-midwives can lash out at each other. Residents can abuse nurses, and nurses can abuse residents. Nurses might choose to make a nurse-midwife's professional life miserable. Doulas backstab and gossip about other doulas.

Why is all this happening? Well, nurses and midwives and residents and doulas do this to each other because they're in pain. They're hurting. They're traumatized. But they also do it because they've internalized their oppression—they see each other as inferior. And sometimes, people do it to identify with or try to assimilate with their oppressor. Or to gain power within systems and teaching institutions—to climb up the ranks, stepping on top of and over their colleagues in a rush to feel more like the people on "top" of the hierarchy.

Does this image, of everyone in the bottom half of the power system fighting each other, instead of banding together to create change, take your breath away? It should! The sad thing is that the second of the two pillars of the system of oppression is *something we're doing to ourselves*. We consciously or subconsciously believe the messages that people in the more dominant group send us—that we're not important. And our own Internalized Oppression helps hold up the existing power structure. How can we possibly create change if we are fighting amongst ourselves and view each other as inferior, worthless, and powerless?

After reading Dr. Love's model, everything started making sense to me. I now understood why it was so difficult to get evidence based care at the hospital where Sarah Wylie and I had both given birth. It also helped me figure out the mystery of why some physicians and midwives (like Michelle) and even nurses who were on the same page as me couldn't seem to make any progress at getting their hospitals to adopt evidence based care practices in labor and delivery. I was thrilled that I had a conceptual framework that could help me understand what was going on.

I also knew that figuring out the *why* might lead to some *solutions*. The power hierarchy seemed so strong—those pillars I've just talked about? They're seemingly set in stone. But I began to dream that maybe, someday, we could lead everyone out of the top-down system and into a circle, where we all valued each other and centered what we do around the family. In fact, at my workshops these days, I usually do just that—I hand the people at the bottom of the hierarchy (the family) some tickets, and say, "These are your tickets out of this top-down system." Then I ask the hospital administrators, lawyers, doctors, nurses, midwives, and others, to leave the top-down line and gather around the family in a circle.

As the circle forms, I always hear an audible, "Awww," coming from the entire group. It's really fun to witness everyone's "Aha" moment happening simultaneously. Right in front of them is the family, the center of everyone's efforts to support them. All the professionals are looking at each other face to face across the circle. "We can see each other now," people say. "I can actually see the family," says the chief obstetrician. "People care about us," says the family. This kind of care system stands in stark contrast to the top-down system they were lined up in minutes before.

And yet, this new system isn't even new. It's been written about for years by physicians, nurses, midwives, and others. It's even got an official name. It's called "Family Centered Care."[114, 115]

You might be wondering, what were those mysterious "tickets out" I handed to the family, that helped them move from the Top-Down System into Family Centered Care? Well, you'll have to wait until the end of this book to find out. It took me years and years after starting Evidence Based Birth before I learned strategies to help individuals dismantle the top-down power hierarchy.

The sun was rising that morning as I sat at my kitchen table, mulling over what I had just read in Dr. Williams's and Dr. Love's research about oppression and power hierarchies. And then, suddenly, one more idea struck me. And that was, I didn't seem to suffer from internalized oppression like so many doulas, nurses, midwives, and women that I knew. I don't know why. Maybe my lack of feeling oppressed came from my privileged upbringing, or the fact that I didn't experience any significant trauma during childhood or adolescence. Maybe it was because my parents let me talk back to them, like an equal, from the time I was a child. Or maybe it came from the rush of empowerment I felt when I gave birth to Henry.

The people at the top of the hierarchy *seemingly* had all the power. But I had this feeling in my gut, that maybe, just maybe, I could do this—I could help create change. I had the confidence, and the knowledge, and the research and writing skills, to make a difference. To help tip the power balance back to where it belonged. To families.

I glanced up from my hand drawn sketch of the power hierarchy as I heard my kids waking up for the day. I leaned back in my chair and smiled. This system was oppressive, but it was also primed for disruption. I just knew it was. And I also knew exactly which one of the Oppressive Factors I wanted to go after. I wanted to focus all my energy on changing culture.

Chapter Six

FRIENDSHIP

I N THE MONTHS AFTER Sarah Wylie had her baby, I went on a huge writing spree. I published blog posts about the Evidence on Diagnosing Gestational Diabetes, Fetal Monitoring, Pushing Positions, and Erythromycin Eye Ointment for Newborns. I published an article called "State of Maternity Care in the U.S.," about how difficult it was to get evidence based care options here. Whenever I felt myself getting upset about Sarah Wylie's experience, I distracted myself by getting lost in the world of research, devouring studies, and translating that research into blog articles for the public.

In these crucial first months of blogging, I also made some decisions that would affect my future in a very big way. One day, while we were folding Clara and Henry's laundry, Dan mentioned that he didn't like one of the blog articles I'd just published.

"You had your opinion in it," he said.

At first, I was offended that my own husband had anything negative to say about my blog! (How dare he?) But then, I realized that he had a point. From then on, I would focus on writing about the evidence, and I would let people form their own opinions. I would not tell them what to do. I also decided to improve the quality of my blog articles by having them peer-reviewed by experts in the field prior to publication.

I also realized, after talking with Dan, that something else felt "off" about the blog. In my first few articles, I'd focused on the evidence on having a "physiologic birth," which is defined as giving birth with your own innate power while avoiding unnecessary medical interventions. Obviously, the information I'd been posting could help people like me, who want to avoid medications during birth. But what about people who *want* or *need* medical interventions during childbirth?

I thought about my sister-in-law Beth. Around the same time that I gave birth to Clara, Beth gave birth by Cesarean to her baby, Will. She was immediately separated from Will—they were forced to recover from surgery in separate rooms, and she described her experience as "cold and clinical." The next time she had a Cesarean with her second son, Owen (a few months before Henry was born), she worked really hard to ensure that she and her baby would be treated better, and that they would get skin-to-skin care as soon as possible after the surgery. She succeeded and had an amazing, family-centered Cesarean birth experience, but it took a lot of advocacy on her part.

I decided that, moving forward, I would cover topics that applied to people who had all kinds of births. This meant I would tackle the evidence on topics like "Skin-to-skin in the Operating Room after a Cesarean," "Group B Strep during

Pregnancy," and other topics that could be useful to anyone, no matter what type of birth you had.

These decisions—making the website relevant to people with all kinds of births, and removing opinions from the articles—would end up catapulting the website to a new level of fandom. People were thrilled to find a website where they could read accurate, unbiased, evidence based information, and that they wouldn't feel "judged" for their decisions or for whatever type of birth they ended up having. You have to understand that during this time period, society was in the height of the "Mommy Wars," where everyone was judging everyone for everybody's parenting choices. So, the fact that I had created a sort of judgment-free zone was particularly appealing.

As the blog became more and more popular, I started to see an increasing number of comments left by people. By chance, the very first comment left under my first blog article came from someone in my hometown named Cristen Pascucci.

Cristen wrote,

> I am so excited about your blog. This is what I would have created if I had had the background, education, and expertise to attempt it! Learning about birth, the myths and the incredible possibilities around it, has been a game-changer for me. Assuming a re-education of the health care profession is not going to take place anytime soon, the truth about birth—which you explore here beautifully—has got to get out to more women.
> ~Cristen

I responded,

> Thank you! I am excited to use my education and
> skills to make a difference in this area. Even when
> the providers hear the evidence, they don't always
> listen. That's why we have to educate consumers
> (i.e. moms). Once consumers demand evidence
> based care, that's when it will happen. It has to do
> with the $$$ signs. I don't think women realize
> how much power they have!

Cristen had a brand-new blog of her own, and I started
posting comments on her blog articles in return. I found out
that she had given birth to her first child, Henry, just 9 days
before I had given birth to my own Henry. And I soon came
to learn her fascinating birth story.

In December 2011, the same time I was due with my Henry,
Cristen was due with her baby Henry. Cristen had worked in
the field of politics and media in Baltimore, Maryland, and
she moved away to be closer to family for when she had her
baby. She originally planned a birth with an obstetrician, but
after she asked too many questions at a prenatal visit, the
obstetrician suggested she switch to a nurse-midwife in the
same practice, and so she did. She was registered to give birth
at a large labor and delivery unit in our town.

After Cristen passed her due date, her midwife started
pressuring her to have a medical labor induction.

Cristen was worried because she didn't want to have an
induction—she wanted the most straightforward, least complicated birth she could have, and she worried that medically
induced contractions might make her more likely to need pain

medication. Cristen's midwife never gave her a medical reason for the induction, but simply told her, "This is what we do."

Cristen wasn't opposed to all inductions—she just didn't understand why they wouldn't give her a good reason she needed one, and she wanted two more days to try to let labor start on its own. Tests on her and the baby kept indicating everyone was healthy, but the pressure from her midwife kept up, and finally Cristen relented on a Thursday, agreeing to schedule an induction for Sunday, but hoping that she would go into labor before then.

Unexpectedly, on Saturday morning, Cristen's phone rang. The midwife had called to tell her they didn't have room for her on the schedule on Sunday after all, that she would need to come in for an induction *that very evening*. Cristen hadn't felt comfortable with the pressure her midwife had been putting on her before, but this was the last straw. She went into action mode—immediately calling her doula and anyone else she thought could help. Her doula, amazingly, was able to point her to a different nurse-midwife, from a different local hospital, who happened to be in the office on a Saturday afternoon and was willing to give Cristen a second opinion right away.

At the office, the new nurse-midwife examined Cristen and explained her options. She told Cristen that she could wait a little bit longer to go into labor on her own, or be induced that night, or have her membranes stripped (a procedure that sometimes makes labor start a little bit earlier) and check back in the next day. After presenting these options as all equally valid choices, the midwife sat back and waited for Cristen to decide what felt best to her. Cristen was stunned. She'd quite simply never had any maternity health care professional treat her like she was a grown-up—laying out the options and leaving her birth decisions entirely up to her.

Cristen ended up choosing to have her membranes stripped once and then wait one more day to see what happened—and she went into labor that night. She had a quick, smooth, unmedicated birth with her new nurse-midwife, at her new hospital. She had switched providers and hospitals on her second-to-last day of pregnancy!

After her birth, Cristen started to process what had happened to her—similar to how I had processed what happened to me. But instead of focusing on the evidence like I did, Cristen had a different point to ponder.

"What," she wondered, "were my *legal rights* in that situation?"

If her first midwife had insisted that she come in for an induction that same day—if Cristen hadn't found a second midwife to support her—could she have been legally forced to be induced? Did she have the right to say no?

Turns out, she did have the right to say no. As an adult human being of sound mind, she had the right to something called informed consent and refusal. Informed consent is both a legal and an ethical concept, and it has two main components—information and consent. *Informed* means you're given complete and accurate information about the pros and cons of all your options, including the option of doing nothing. The *consent* part of the equation means that you are free to say "yes" or "no," without pressure, coercion, or threats of force. Refusal of medical treatment is a right of all people, rooted in the constitution and human rights principles. It means you can say "no" to medical treatment even if it is life-saving for you or someone else (for example, an organ transplant from you that would let another person live longer).[116, 117]

Now, if you ask a random stranger, "Who is the legal authority in the labor and delivery room?" many people might say, "The doctor." Although the doctor is viewed as an authority figure by many people, he or she is not the legal authority over the woman's body or baby. The person who is giving birth is the one who has the right to say "yes" or "no" to any medical care offered to them.

Nobody can tell someone who's about to give birth what they can and cannot do. Health care professionals can advise the pregnant person—they can recommend a certain course of action—but they cannot force it on the patient. And if they use pressure or coercion or lies or bullying to get a client to comply with their wishes, then they are violating the ethical principle of autonomy, which is defined as the right to bodily integrity. Some care providers, when they violate patient autonomy, might even do so in such a way that they commit obstetric violence—defined as when care providers exercise inappropriate control over birthing people's bodies and choices through the use of abuse, coercion, or disrespect.[118]

I was fascinated by Cristen's story and by her passion for the human and legal rights of birthing families in the health care system. She was extremely intelligent, loved to write (just like me), and had different and more expansive ways of thinking about childbirth than anybody I'd ever met. She lived just a few miles from me. She had a son named Henry, for goodness' sake! And, like me, she had recently made it her life's mission to help change the childbirth care system. So much so that she didn't return to work after her Henry was born, and instead volunteered her time—working full-time unpaid—to help women who were facing difficult birth circumstances.

She connected them with lawyers and talked them through their options when they were facing disrespectful or non-evidence based care.

In August 2012, about eight months after our Henrys were born, I invited Cristen to come to a peer-to-peer support group for mothers with babies so that we could meet in real life for the first time. We and the Henrys hit it off immediately! We started making playdates to get together more often. Pretty much 100% of the time (Dan can vouch for this), our conversation would turn to birth, how messed up the health care system was, and our dreams for creating change.

One day, the Henrys were crawling around my basement playroom together, putting every toy they could find into their mouths, and I mentioned to Cristen that I'd just met someone online named Dawn Thompson, who had started a non-profit called ImprovingBirth.org. Dawn's non-profit was hosting a nationwide rally on Labor Day (get it? Labor Day?). The event was called "Rally to Improve Birth," and they were looking for a volunteer to help them write a press release. I suggested Cristen reach out to Dawn, since Cristen had public relations expertise and wanted to get involved in birth at the national level.

Next thing I know, both Cristen and I were knee deep helping Dawn plan for a nationwide rally. The rally was supposed to take place in front of over one hundred hospitals across the U.S., where families would hold up signs on the sidewalk, advocating for evidence based, respectful care. I was thrilled to have found people who were as excited about this cause as I was, and I threw myself into the effort, using my spare time in the evenings and weekends to help Dawn create infographics for social media, and providing Cristen with the statistics she needed for press releases and other materials.

On the Friday before the 2012 Labor Day Rally, I was sitting in a meeting at my college of nursing. It was my first meeting as chairperson of the undergraduate admissions committee. I had just opened the meeting and welcomed everyone, when suddenly, I started seeing spots in my right eye. White dots floated around everywhere, but only on my right side.

I felt nauseated and dazed. I explained what was happening, and my coworkers told me to go home. About 30 minutes after walking into my house, I was hit with the worst headache of my life.

I had never had an aura before (the visual symptoms before a migraine), and I had also never sought emergency care for a migraine before. This time, though, the pain was so bad I thought I was going to die, so I went to the Emergency Room. I was vomiting and couldn't keep any medications down. I continued to suffer from severe migraine pain for the next eight days—having to make one more visit to the ER, and two visits to urgent care.

On Sunday, the night before the Rally, I lay in my dark bedroom, unable to eat, sleep, or think. Cristen called, and I forced myself to answer. We needed to talk with Dawn about last-minute details about the Rally to Improve Birth. My eyes closed, ice pack on my forehead, I gave them a few tips about the research on childbirth for the next day's Rally.

That week, I learned a hard lesson, and it was one that would be reinforced repeatedly over the next several years: When I get a migraine, I have to take care of myself. This was so frustrating, because taking care of a moderate-to-severe migraine generally means lying in the dark doing nothing. You can't read, you can't write, you can't talk, and you can barely think. And if you have learned anything about me from reading this book so far, you might have guessed that I am NOT the kind of person who can just lie around doing nothing.

I was on a mission—I was determined to make evidence based care the norm for childbirth. How could I fulfill my mission if I was having so much pain? And I had a lot of pain—I had about 15 migraines per month, or about half of my waking and sleeping time spent in pain. I figured a way to cope, and that was to use every minute of my spare time when I felt good or halfway decent. It was critical to be super-productive, because I never knew when the next severe migraine would strike.

At the start of the fall 2012 semester, the stress was building. There was my job (which had ramped up with the beginning of classes and my newly funded grant), my blog, my husband, my kids, and the rest of my extended family. Plus, I had to get meals on the table, manage our household, and try to get some sleep. And, about half the time, I was in pain. One night, before going to bed, exhausted, I made the mistake of checking Facebook. Right then, I discovered that a public critique had been written about me online.

I saw the headline and my heart started racing. I had been struggling with trolls who had been posting comments on my blog, but it was *my* blog, so I had been able to delete and moderate comments as needed. But this was an actual article, posted online, written by a retired physician (a former obstetrician), targeting me by name.

"Oh no," I thought. "Why did I check Facebook right before bedtime? Never, ever again."

I could not fall asleep that night. The thought that someone I didn't know would write such words about me frightened me. I couldn't even bring myself to read the article in its entirety. The next morning, exhausted after a sleepless night, I asked both Dan and Cristen to read the article and paraphrase it for me.

Dan read it and told me at once that he thought it was ridiculous.

Cristen wrote me a reassuring email:

"Okay, I just read it in depth. If you want to read it, don't be anxious. It's so stupid, I think you would just laugh. It has references to Rebecca Dekker, Decker, and Becker. It's a lot of bluster, illogical arguments, and sarcasm with an odd 'Orwellian' theme that doesn't even make sense. The article title, 'New website, Evidence Based Birth, suffers from a shocking lack of evidence,' is a shot across your bow. So, what? Based on what I've seen, I'd ask who reads this woman, and why would you care what she writes? It's a joke. She's like a paper dragon. Ignore, ignore, ignore. Don't waste your time on it, because no one who matters will."

Relieved, I decided to agree with Cristen. Moving forward, I would ignore this writer's critique, as well as the trolling comments on my blog. And it's a good thing I had this policy, because over the next few months, it would happen again! Another article was written about me by this same physician, this one entitled, "Rebecca Dekker's 'Evidence Based Birth': you can put lipstick on a pig, but it's still a pig," complete with a cartoon image of my website as a pig wearing bright red lipstick and red high heels. I was horrified that when you Googled my name the third result (temporarily) was the article she'd written about me and my website being a pig with lipstick. But despite my horror, I did have to chuckle, because I have never—not even once in my life—worn lipstick. Or high heels.

Meanwhile, in the comments section of my blog, I had to delete more and more trolling comments, increasingly frustrated at the time I had to spend dealing with this crowd. Did these people not have a life? Because I certainly did! Who has time for this? Some of the comments were outright disrespectful and crazy, so I could delete them immediately, but other trolls used a slightly more roundabout way to get their first comments approved before they started attacking me with subsequent comments. One person in particular, who used the screen name "Captain Obvious," would try to lure me into a trap using a philosophical argument style. He would make some comments that seemed initially pleasant and respectful, but intended to ruffle my feathers, and then *bam* make statements like, "You're going to be the cause of a lot of dead babies."

By this point, I'd had enough of ignoring. It was time to move beyond ignoring, to building a wall, and to not letting these people use the comments section of my website to spread their toxic ideas. I happened to see an article on Popular Science about why they were turning off their comments section on their blog.[119] They mentioned a new research study showing that comment sections are detrimental to scientific blog articles—and well, it was only one study, but it was enough of an excuse for me![120] I turned off the comments section, and almost instantly, my quality of life improved and my stress level went down.

These encounters taught me a lot about the field of childbirth.

Never before, in my previous area of research (cardiovascular science), had I ever encountered troll-like behavior. In the cardiovascular field, there was an expectation of professionalism, respect for patient autonomy, and collaboration. In fact, that same fall, I had traveled to the American Heart Association Scientific Sessions, where I won a new investigator award, and I was struck by the collaboration between all the different professions—between nurses and doctors and bench scientists and social workers and patient advocates. In contrast, when you ventured into the field of childbirth, there seemed to be very little collaboration between professions—there was no unifying conference, and all the different professions were educated in silos. Pregnant parents, or "patients," or "patient advocates," were not visibly present at any of the obstetric conferences—they were not considered to be part of the health care "team." Furthermore, there was a very vocal group who believed that women should not be free to make *any* choices about the care that they receive during their baby's birth. The thought was that women should just lie back and do as the doctor says.

The judgment and the vitriol and the lack of respect for bodily autonomy were disturbing, to say the least.

There came a point toward the end of that first year of blogging when Cristen and I both felt like we were screaming into a void. It seemed like an uphill battle—the longer we immersed ourselves into the field of childbirth, the more we were exposed to the depth and breadth of the problem. We knew we were following in the footsteps of strong women who'd been speaking up, for generations, about the lack of respectful care in childbirth. But among the general public, nobody seemed to be talking about birth trauma, or the lack of evidence based care, in any kind of organized way. No one seemed to care.

It was a good thing we could commiserate with each other—otherwise I probably would have given up. Cristen and I began to call each other on a daily basis to talk about what we could do to create change. We decided to team up to write an editorial for our local newspaper. Cristen began scheming about how she could use her prior experience as a public relations professional to get birth trauma into the national news media.

Thankfully, with the free time that I gained by saying "goodbye" to the comments section of my website, I began to relax a little bit toward the end of that semester. Clara had just turned four and, in addition to going to preschool and playing piano, she loved dressing up in princess costumes, singing, and twirling around for what seemed like hours in our living room. Henry, almost a year old now, had the biggest, goofiest smile, and was starting to walk and climb up onto chairs and tables. Some weekends, Cristen would bring her Henry over to play, and together, the two boys would get into everything—the dishwasher, the stereo equipment, the (empty) fireplace.

Curious one day about how many people were visiting my website, I checked the analytics and discovered that people were reading my articles from all over the world! Although most of my readers were from the U.S., website visitors were coming from all over—from Australia and Afghanistan to Vietnam and Zimbabwe!

I was astounded and thrilled and anxious all at the same time. When I first started, the intention was to maybe eventually reach 10 or 12 people *total* . . . so, I hadn't felt the need to tell my employers about it. A few of my coworkers knew what I was doing, but none of my supervisors. Now that I was getting so much traffic, I would have to disclose my blog and find out if the university was okay with me blogging on my time off. I was nervous about what they might think.

I requested an appointment with the dean of my college. A week later, as we sat in her administrative suite, she looked thoughtfully at me while I told her everything that had happened leading up to the start of the blog. I shared my two birth stories. I talked about how I'd been collecting the evidence and making handouts. I told her how I just wanted to publish literature reviews, but I was getting all this traffic, and now the blog was becoming bigger than I ever imagined. Then I sat back and waited anxiously for her response.

When I recall this moment, I remember that the dean smiled. She told me she was proud of me and she had a feeling I was destined to do great things.

What happened next is a bit fuzzy in my memory. I can't remember if she said, it, or if I said it. But regardless, one of us brought up the fact that the hospital side of the university might see my blog as a direct threat to their way of doing things. They probably wouldn't notice me for a while. But eventually, if my blog became popular enough, they would. How could we protect me from retaliation?

I had known from the start that my blog might irritate some people. They might view it as a critique of traditions and routines in labor and delivery. But before that meeting, I had never considered that I might be seen as a threat, that the hospital might retaliate against me—that I might need *protecting*.

Over the next few weeks, with the help of university staff and their lawyers, I formulated a plan. First, I was advised that I should never mention the university by name on my website, so that the blog would not appear to be affiliated with the university in any way. I also knew this would help prevent the hospital administrators from realizing I worked at the same university as them, so if they stumbled across the blog, they wouldn't put two and two together, at least not for a while. I was pretty sure I hadn't mentioned the blog in my first meeting with those administrators, and I was thankful I'd kept my mouth shut at the time.

Second, I would work on the blog during my personal time, so that the blog would not be considered part of my faculty role—it would be part of my private life. This had an added benefit of meaning that the content on the blog was my own private intellectual property. Also, any time I was interviewed by a reporter or anybody else from the media about birth-related topics, I would call myself, "Rebecca Dekker, PhD, RN, faculty member at a research-intensive university in the southeast," effectively erasing the university credentials from my bio in those situations. This would allow me to speak freely with the media whenever I was contacted for an interview.

But did I *really* have "freedom of speech?" Was that even possible when you worked for an institution? With my new protection plan, I did feel better about my situation. But I still worried about the possibility of censure or even—worst case scenario—losing my job. From now on, I would have to tread very carefully.

Chapter Seven

SURPRISE

B EFORE THE END OF THE YEAR, both Cristen and I received an invitation to join the board of the non-profit ImprovingBirth.org—the same organization we had already helped out with during the Labor Day Rally. These were "working" board positions, in which we would need to volunteer time to move the organization forward.

I was excited about the work ImprovingBirth.org was doing, and I thought my work-life balance was doing okay at the moment, so I said yes.

Cristen, the new Vice President of the Board, and myself, the Secretary, suddenly found ourselves in the thick of non-profit work, which involved a lot of email correspondence and many phone meetings about creating change at the national level.

Suddenly, right around the same time I started this new volunteer position, we began having problems with childcare.

Briana, our wonderful nanny who had been with us for two-and-a-half years—and had even been present at Henry's home birth—got married and moved to Florida. I didn't think it would be that big of a deal to replace her.

But after Briana left, we hired nanny after nanny after nanny, and none of them came close to matching how Briana had become part of our family. Also, none of the new nannies lasted more than a few months. When we had a nanny in place, they weren't always reliable—calling in for illness and other excuses, usually with no notice. Every time one of our nannies quit, or was fired, I had to go through a lengthy process of posting the job, going through applications, doing several rounds of interviews, and checking references. Then, when we finally found someone, I had to work from home for about a week, orienting the new person to our kids' routines. Because my job as an assistant professor had more flexibility, and Dan had strict 9-to-5 work hours where he had to be physically present at his job, the responsibility of finding and training each babysitter—as well as covering for them when they inevitably called in sick without notice—fell solely to me.

The next spring, I sent an email apologizing to Dawn and Cristen, because I felt I hadn't been doing a fair share of the volunteer work at ImprovingBirth.org.

I wrote, "This was a bad week for me because my babysitter was sick Mon-Wed, and so I've been behind on regular work stuff. I am leaving Saturday morning for vacation—Dan and I are renting a house on the beach without the kids. I am simultaneously excited to go but afraid to leave them behind. I'll be back the following weekend."

Cristen's response? Three words.

"Don't get preggers."

In the end, Dan and I had a wonderful vacation. It was our first trip without kids in several years, and we enjoyed the time we had to refresh and reconnect. However, even though we were together in such a beautiful place, I couldn't stop thinking about evidence based care, and how I wished I could help more families attain it. One morning, as I sat on a patio overlooking the ocean, barefoot, with a cool breeze on my face, I sketched out an outline of a course I wanted to create to teach families about evidence based care. I so wanted to be able to teach and mentor families. I also wanted families to get the kind of care they wanted, without resistance from hospital staff. But this dream seemed far out of reach.

Suddenly, I thought about a quote I'd recently read from George Bernard Shaw.[121] It was corny, but it stuck out in my mind:

"You see things; and you say 'Why?' But I dream things that never were; and I say, 'Why not?'"

I headed back to work the next week, refreshed, hopeful, and rested, but—I'll admit it—a little bit reluctant to return to the real world. The fact was, even though I had distracted myself from the local situation by volunteering at ImprovingBirth.org and writing for Evidence Based Birth, I continued to be frustrated by the lack of evidence based care in my home town. The stories of people who received bad care during childbirth at some of the nearby hospitals seemed never-ending. By now, it had been nearly five years since Clara's birth and I was still hearing from families and doulas that evidence based care was extremely hard to come by at most hospitals in my state, if not downright impossible to obtain.

After careful thought, I decided to do two things. First, I asked Cristen if she would help me host an official Rally to Improve Birth in our city in the upcoming September of 2013. We recruited a team of seven community members to work on this (including Sarah Wylie!) as a group effort. Cristen was assigned to public relations and getting media attention, while I was in charge of logistics—finding a rally site, getting the appropriate city permits, and figuring out how to encourage local families to attend.

Second, I decided to organize a letter-writing campaign in which mothers would write letters to administrators at my university health care system. Sarah Wylie volunteered immediately. She composed a thoughtful, well-written letter about her experience giving birth there (including how difficult it was to get intermittent auscultation), and sent it to four executives, including the executive vice president of the entire health care system, whose email I procured for her.

The following day, she got this response:

"I apologize for your inconveniences. I have asked the appropriate people to address your concerns."

She never heard from them again.

After that, I was discouraged, but I refused to give up. Just like before, I turned my energy toward my Circle of Influence. I did as much as I could behind the scenes—reaching out to consumers who had given birth at my university, encouraging them to speak out about their concerns, planning the rally, and continuing to publish research articles at Evidence Based Birth, including two articles that went viral: "The Evidence on Induction or C-section for Big Baby" and "The Evidence on Failure to Progress."

Later that spring, I was having a particularly rough time. I was exhausted from work. Also, I was worried I had come down with a stomach bug, because as I lay on the couch, listening to Dan make dinner for the kids, all of a sudden I felt kind of queasy.

"Ugh," I thought, "A stomach bug is the last thing I need right now."

Or was it a stomach bug?

Could I possibly be . . . pregnant? It was possible, although unlikely. A few months back, I had decided to go off of my birth control, to see if that would reduce my migraine frequency (one of many unsuccessful medication adjustments I'd make over the years). I was still breastfeeding Henry, who was just a little over a year old, and when you counted my 40-week pregnancy with him, I hadn't had a period in about two years.

That night, I mentioned to Dan that maybe I would stop by the drug store and get a pregnancy test the next day. Just to check.

On the way to work, I purchased a test and stuck it in my backpack. As soon as I got to work, I unlocked my office, dumped my stuff on my desk, grabbed the test, and headed straight for the bathroom.

As I urinated on the test, it turned positive.

Immediately.

I couldn't believe it. It had taken so much time and effort to get pregnant with Clara and Henry . . . and here I was, with a surprise pregnancy, and no idea when I had gotten pregnant!

For the next 8 hours, I kept my pregnancy a secret. I didn't call Dan. I didn't tell anybody.

As I walked to the university café later that day for lunch, I basked in the knowledge of this child who I hadn't anticipated, but who would soon come to be. The hallways were crowded as people bustled past me. There was the potential for new life growing inside of me, and none of these people knew. It was thrilling to carry such a big surprise, and hold it just to myself.

I got home that afternoon and Dan didn't ask me anything about the test. As we were cleaning up supper and he was loading the dishwasher, I casually leaned against the counter.

"Sooo . . . I'm pregnant."

"You're what??" Dan exclaimed.

"I'm pregnant!"

"But what, when . . . wait, what?" He went on, dumbfounded.

"I have no idea when it happened," I said. "I don't even have a clue when the estimated due date would be."

It turns out Dan had thought for sure the test had been negative—because I hadn't called him right away that morning. For once, and the only time in our lives, we got to revel in the newness of a surprise pregnancy.

A few weeks later, it was time to share the news with everyone. The first person I told, aside from Dan, was Karen (good news, she could attend our birth!). My sister was not surprised—having been through a difficult pregnancy herself by now, she could spot my morning sickness a mile away. Our parents were thrilled. My coworkers and boss at work were excited for me.

And I *think* Cristen was happy, but knowing her, I guarantee you she said, "Oh, no, what are we going to do now?" after we got off the phone.

Except you'd need to substitute an expletive for the word "no."

In May, I had an ultrasound to date the pregnancy. Because I hadn't had a period, we really had no solid idea of when the baby was due. Based on when my morning sickness symptoms had started, my best guess was a due date of December 20. But the ultrasound said that my due date was December 12—a discrepancy of 8 days. I was happy about the earlier due date—that meant we'd have our new baby by Christmas. I had absolutely loved having a holiday baby when Henry was born—it was the best gift ever. A cute newborn to dress up in snuggly red pajamas and cuddle with on Christmas Eve? Yes, please!

My pregnancy forced my hand in several matters. The migraine severity I'd had with my earlier pregnancies returned with a vengeance. Day after day, night after night, I suffered from pain in my head and neck. I forced myself to go to work, and Dan bought me a used recliner from Craigslist for my university office—hauling it into the building and up the elevator to my office on the fourth floor. The recliner was there in case the pain got so severe that I couldn't drive home (there was nowhere at work for me to lie down). When I got home from work each night, I would collapse on the couch, or in bed, with a towel shielding my eyes from light and an ice pack on my head.

Dan took on the bulk of parenting duties during this pregnancy—cooking the kids' meals, reading them books, tucking them in at bedtime. By the end of my pregnancy, Henry, nearly two years old, cried if I tried to tuck him in—he asked for Daddy. He'd grown so used to me being out of commission that he didn't want me anymore.

My whole life I'd dreamed of having a large family with four or five children. But this level of pain and physical suffering, and the fact that my children had to go without their mommy every night, was enough to force me to admit that this was it—we were done with three. This was the end of my big family dreams.

The other thing this pregnancy made me do was cull my to-do list. I realized that volunteering my time at ImprovingBirth.org was not something I could do anymore. The reality was, I had no extra time! The time I did have needed to be spent working on my tenure-track faculty position, taking care of my family, and writing articles for the blog at Evidence Based Birth. I called Dawn and gave her my notice—she wasn't surprised; she knew I was spread too thin.

However, I had one volunteer commitment I wanted to finish—I wanted to work with the local team to organize the Rally in September. The Rally was super important to me, because I thought it would be a way we could get our message in the media, and as a result, to hospital administrators. It was critical to get the word out that families wanted more options than were currently offered in local hospitals.

My decision to help with the Rally was reinforced when a nursing student came to my office upset by what she'd seen in our university's labor and delivery unit. The student told me that an Amish woman had come to birth her seventh baby in the hospital. Normally, Amish women give birth at home with midwives (at times, Karen attended their births), but this mother was here, birthing at an academic medical center, because she had a non-pregnancy-related medical condition that needed to be operated on a few days after the baby was born.

The patient, instructed to labor in bed, had said to the nurse and nursing student, "I'm scared. I don't know how to give birth in a bed. I've never done it that way before. I've only ever given birth standing up."

The labor nurse said, "Don't worry. You'll lie on your back, and we'll put your feet in stirrups, and we'll deliver your baby for you."

The nursing student froze. She didn't know what to say or do. All she could do was come to me afterward, shaken.

This student knew, instinctively, that it was a human right to be able to choose your position when giving birth, and she had just witnessed her preceptor, an experienced nurse, take the patient's choice away. And not just any patient—but a client from the plain community, whose cultural practices included unmedicated, upright birth. Why was this done, even though it wasn't culturally sensitive for the patient? Because the culture of the *unit* dictated that patients must give birth in bed, on their backs, with their legs spread apart and their feet either in stirrups or being held up in the air by the nurses (this position is also known as the lithotomy position).

As the years passed, I would hear about many similar situations taking place at my university's hospital. What people told me was that if women wanted to push in upright positions, they were sometimes allowed to do so for a little bit. But as soon as the baby's head was about to emerge, the woman would be pressured to get into the lithotomy position for the actual emergence of the baby's head, with doctors and nurses usually citing the "safety" of the baby for the reason of the position change.

But the real reason they enforced the lithotomy position? It was more familiar and comfortable for the doctors and nurses. It was likely the only way they knew how to "deliver" a baby. Believe it or not, I was told that the nurses, residents, and obstetricians there thought that giving birth in an upright position, like I did with Henry, was thought of as giving birth "upside down!"

The Rally ended up being a huge success! We rented a big park downtown with great visibility, had perfect weather, more than a dozen sponsors, raised thousands of dollars for ImprovingBirth.org nationally, got articles in the newspaper and segments on the local television news shows, and nearly 400 people turned out to show their support for evidence based maternity care. Dan came and helped staff the bounce house full of toddlers, and Clara helped me hold handmade signs by the street saying, "Evidence Based Care" and "We Can Do Better!" One nearby hospital, already supportive of evidence based options, even had a table exhibiting at the rally—advertising the fact that they provided water immersion, intermittent auscultation, and midwifery care.

To me, the crowds were validation that families in our town desperately wanted evidence based options for childbirth. Sadly, though, with the exception of the one hospital that had an exhibit table at our rally, none of the other hospitals chose to attend. We'd invited them, but never received a response. In my opinion, the cultural norms there were too powerful. We wouldn't be seeing change for a while.

In the meantime, though, my Circle of Influence was growing. I got good news from the U.S. Patent and Trademark Office—I found out that my application was approved, and I was now the official owner of a trademark: "Evidence Based Birth®"! I also started an email newsletter and several thousand people signed up right away!

Whenever I thought about my situation, it was hard to believe how much the blog had grown in just a year and a half. I had so many people following my work now that they wouldn't even fit in a school gymnasium if we all got together in real life! I got giddy just thinking about the power of what we could do if all of us were advocating for evidence based care at the same time!

Although I was happy about the excitement my blog was generating, it also made me a little nervous, because, as you know, I'm an introvert. I didn't want people to find out too much about my private life. I didn't mind writing about the evidence to my audience, but I would not talk about my personal life—that was where I drew the line.

So, naturally, I hid my pregnancy from the public. Nobody, outside my family, close friends, and coworkers, knew I was having a third baby. To those of you who think it is impossible to hide a pregnancy on social media, I'm here to tell you it can be done!

My due date in December 2013 arrived quickly. I'd been seeing Karen on the normal prenatal schedule—every 4 weeks in the beginning, then every 2 weeks, then weekly starting at 36 weeks. At 40 weeks, on December 12, I was feeling good, but there were no signs that labor would be starting anytime soon. I was discouraged, but determined to have a home birth, and I knew I needed to avoid the university hospital—the only one covered by my insurance. I also knew that, if I went in for an induction, chances were slim to none that I would be able to get the other things I wanted on my birth plan. Thankfully, being a third-time mother, with two prior successful vaginal births, it was highly unlikely that I would need hospital care.

But with each passing day, there was still no sign of labor.

On December 19, at 41 weeks of pregnancy, Karen and I decided to get prenatal testing to monitor the pregnancy, and we also discussed the possibility that maybe, just maybe, the dating ultrasound hadn't been accurate. It was hard to know for sure. She said that based on my physical exam and how I looked the last time I was pregnant, with Henry, that I didn't *look* 41 weeks pregnant right now—I looked more like 40 weeks. Ultrasounds at 11 to 14 weeks, like the one I'd had, are supposed to be very accurate. But research shows that the true due date could be as much as 11 days earlier or later than an 11- to 14-week ultrasound's estimation.[122] We were both questioning if December 12 was correct. Still, several times that week, I went to a local doctor for some prenatal testing, just to make sure everything was okay with my baby. The tests showed all was well.

On December 20, I picked up the phone and called my mom. I wanted to find out when all of my various siblings and their family would be heading to town to celebrate Christmas with us. There are six of us siblings, and along with spouses and children, it's a big crowd.

"They arrive tomorrow," she said.

"Okay, and when does the last person leave?" I asked.

"Hmm, looks like the last one leaves on December 29."

I immediately knew that my body wouldn't go into labor while my family was in town. Not with everyone hanging around, watching my every step, asking me repeatedly, "Has labor started yet?" "Are you feeling anything?" "When is that baby coming?"

Christmas Eve came. I still hadn't given up hope of having my Christmas baby—maybe labor would start tonight? No.

Christmas Day? No.

Finally, on December 28, three days after Christmas, I felt nauseated and threw up once, then experienced mild contractions. They were real, and they came regularly. I called Karen, and she came over to assess me. But after a few hours, I fell asleep, the contractions stopped, and Karen went home. The next day, one of our kids started throwing up, and I realized that my nausea the day before was not a sign of labor—it was a mild stomach bug.

On December 29, I felt better—my stomach felt fine—but at this point I was desperate for labor to begin. I did not want to go to the university hospital.

Although waiting for labor to start on its own is a reasonable option, I also knew that research shows that, when you have a healthy pregnancy, electively inducing labor at 39 weeks or later is *also* a reasonable option.[123,124] Which option you choose, according to researchers, is highly dependent on your unique clinical situation and your goals, values, and preferences.

Even though by this point I would have preferred to do something to medically induce my labor, I felt that if I went to the hospital and requested a medical labor induction at the documented "42 weeks and 4 days," the hospital staff—the obstetricians and the nurses—would have *flipped out*. In my imagination, I pictured myself walking in there, immediately being labeled as a problem patient, and treated accordingly. In their culture, they would have never "let" someone go past 42 weeks, even though my due date was in question. Even though research at the time showed that waiting for spontaneous labor at 39, 40, 41, *or* 42 weeks* is a reasonable option for someone with a healthy pregnancy.[124,125]

I also had heard by this point that the nurses and doctors knew that I was the blogger behind Evidence Based Birth® (EBB), and that I wasn't the most liked person on that unit. So, afraid of how they might treat me, I made the decision to wait for labor to start on its own. But that didn't mean I couldn't try some "natural" induction techniques at home!

After supper that night, I sat down at my desk in the basement and reviewed research on ways to naturally induce labor. I was composing an email to send to a local acupuncturist, to see if she could give me a treatment to help induce labor, when all of a sudden, a strong pressure wave gripped me.

"Dan," I yelled up the stairs, "It's starting!"

Within a half-hour, Karen and her assistant were at our house, setting up the birth supplies and tub in the nursery. Dan tucked the kids in bed upstairs, and then ran back down to help me with Hypnobabies® cues and scripts. Just like last time, with Henry, my birthing time was easy—much easier and way more pleasant than a migraine. I didn't feel pain, just pressure. I had practiced my self-hypnosis skills daily for the past few months, and it was paying off.

---

*Research continues to emerge on the benefits and risks of inducing labor at different time points. New research indicates that induction at 41 weeks can help reduce stillbirths (especially for first-time mothers) without increasing harm. See ebbirth.com/inducingduedates for the latest info.

Midnight passed, and I got in the tub. A little before 2 a.m., I heard Karen tell Dan that she was worried I was getting tired. The last few weeks had been exhausting for me, and I was getting sleepy. She asked my permission to check my cervix, just to see if I was ready to push.

"Rebecca!" she said with surprise. "The head is right there! If you push a few times, your baby will be born!"

She then turned to our doula, and said, "Quick! Go wake up Clara! If she wants to see this birth, she better get down here fast, because Rebecca's babies fly out!"

We'd had no idea I was on the verge of giving birth! I was in the same position I'd been last time when I gave birth to Henry— on my knees, with arms and head resting on the side of the soft inflatable tub. I gathered up my courage, and gently bore down once. Then I took a deep breath and breathed my baby out.

And so, in less than three minutes of pushing, Susanna was born. Like her big brother Henry, Susie was born underwater. Also like her brother Henry, she was exactly 9 pounds, 2 ounces. And big sister Clara made it there just in time to see her sibling born.

The newborn assessment was just as joyful as last time, although we were all a bit sleepier, due to it being the wee hours of the morning. Five-year-old Clara, her mouth scrunched in concentration, cut her little sister's cord, then promptly flopped down and fell asleep in bed with us. Henry never woke up— he slept upstairs through the whole birth!

Karen and her assistant carefully examined Susie.

According to Karen's physical exam, Susie's gestational age was approximately 41 weeks.

She was not 42 weeks and 4 days like the dating ultra-sound had said. My instinct—that the ultrasound-calculated due date was off—was correct all along.

Susie's pregnancy was an exhausting experience for me. The birth itself was easy, but the long wait for labor to begin, the uncertainty of my due date, the stress of the holidays, and the many months of migraines, had worn me down. And to be honest, I was saddened by my situation. How could it be that I felt so afraid of going to the hospital affiliated with my university, when an induction is what I would have preferred in hindsight? Was that my fault? Or theirs? Or a combination of both?

Susie's birth also affirmed that I was on the right track with my blog—*this is what I was meant to do*. By now, I knew that it *was* possible for hospitals to provide evidence based care and respect patient autonomy. I'd heard accounts from professionals and parents about a handful of hospitals across the country that seemed like ideal places to give birth. Freestanding birth centers, which have excellent outcomes,[126] were also scattered across the U.S. But no freestanding birth centers were available in my state (the last attempt to open a birth center had ended with the three nearest hospitals fighting in court—and winning—to prevent the birth center from opening). Even local hospitals with better reputations had limitations, including unpredictable care and restrictive policies. A nursing student had told me that she'd witnessed a doctor cut a forced episiotomy on a first-time mom during an uncomplicated vaginal birth. The mother was pushing nicely and her perineum was gradually stretching over the baby's head. The doctor, impatient and tired of waiting, let out a big sigh, grabbed the scissors, and—*snip*—cut the woman's vagina, just like that. Without even asking. And this was at the "good" hospital in our area!

I knew I was fortunate in that I had the option to "opt out" of the system and have a home birth—not only did I have the financial resources to pay a midwife out of pocket, but I also had the desire and the support to give birth at home, physiologically. In contrast, most people I knew (including most of the people I care about in my life) will probably give birth in hospitals, either because they have risk factors that make a home birth less safe, or a medical need for interventions, or a desire for pain medications, or because their insurance will only cover care in a hospital, or because they simply want to be in a hospital.

The whole situation with Susie's birth made me wonder: What would it take to turn things around? To make hospitals more predictable places to get high-quality care during childbirth? To make all those things I loved about home birth—the family-centered care, the privacy, the autonomous midwifery care, the labor support, the non-pharmacologic comfort measures—easily accessible in hospitals? And what would it take to make freestanding birth centers available to families who wanted that option?

In the meantime, how many other families out there were, like me, nervous about seeking care at a hospital? Would there ever be anything I could do to fix that?

Chapter Eight

WOKE

THANKFULLY, AS SOON AS Susie was born, I felt amazing. The migraines lifted and, like last time, I felt a surge of energy. With the pain gone, I was able to become a better mom to Clara and Henry again. They were so adorable, always asking to cuddle with Susie. I was excited and feeling incredibly lucky that I would get 12 weeks paid leave at home with my three little ones—something that was unheard of among most of my family and friends (most of whom went back to work at 4 to 6 weeks postpartum).

I was feeling so inspired that I published a big blog article before I went back to work, called "Evidence on Vitamin K for Newborns." Surprisingly, the article was so controversial that the website kept crashing due to the traffic demand on the servers. Dan and I had to scramble to find a new web host that could handle the traffic, and it was a week before our website was back online.

I went back to work at the end of March, mulling over the public's reaction to the Vitamin K article. I hadn't thought an article about a vitamin would be a big deal. But, apparently, there was a lot of misinformation out there on the Internet, and people had been misled into believing myths about Vitamin K being harmful (it isn't). I'd also discovered that part of the controversy was related to the fact that some people thought I should only write about the evidence for *avoiding* interventions. They were upset that I'd written that evidence clearly supports the use of Vitamin K—an intervention—for newborns!

One midwife from another country was so angry with me that she figured out where I worked, called my university, got an administrative assistant on the phone, and yelled at her about how I was a horrible person and a "tyrant." She was mad that there wasn't a comments section on my website—that makes me a tyrant?

But, as Dan reminded me, people needed to learn that I wasn't out there to promote any one type of birth. I was, as he said, "on the side of the evidence." In the end, this position— being on the side of the evidence—solidified my following. A lot of my readers were relieved I didn't have a secret agenda, that I really was just there to serve them by democratizing the evidence and making it available to everyone. And so, my audience grew.

As Susie's first year progressed, Dan and I continued to experience difficulties with childcare. We had to hire a new nanny (our fifth) at the end of my maternity leave in March, and when August rolled around, she quit. With the beginning of the academic year looming over me, I gritted my teeth, sat down at my desk at home, and posted another nanny ad. As usual, I got responses right away and began the screening process. One candidate in particular stood out to me. She wanted to leave daycare work to spend more time with families. During her interview, she sat on the floor and played with Susie, seemingly enamored with my youngest child, who was now about 8 months old.

I thought, "Maybe this is it! Maybe she's the one who will finally work out!"

This sixth nanny started the next week. I was excited for her first day, and I planned to work from home so I could show her everything around the house and answer her questions. School was still out for the summer, so all three kids were around.

The morning seemed to go well, but, at 1 p.m., the new nanny walked into my home office.

She said, "I don't think I want to work for you. This isn't the right fit for me."

I said, "Wait . . . what's going on? What's wrong?"

"You know what? I really only want to take care of babies. I could see myself caring for your baby, she's adorable, but older children? Like a five-year-old and two-year-old? That's just not my thing."

"Wait . . . what?" I thought. "Then why did you take this job, when I have an infant, a two-year-old, *and* a five-year-old?"

She packed up her bag and left. I sat on the floor and cried. It was just too much. How could I do everything I wanted to do—my faculty job and my blog—when I couldn't get help with my kids? Was it impossible to be a working mom? I felt an ache in my heart—one I'm sure many parents have felt—when you're in that horrible dilemma of trying to figure out how to make a living while finding affordable, reliable care for beloved children.

For the seventh time in two years, we were stuck without anybody to watch our children the next day.

This sixth nanny—the one who quit on her first day—this was the straw that broke my camel's back. I called Dan. He answered, and, sobbing, I told him what had happened.

"Hold on," he said. "I'm coming home."

A few minutes later, I heard the back door open and Dan's footsteps as he walked toward the nursery. He knelt on the floor next to me and I melted into his arms. Dan has always been my other half, my best friend in the whole world. He is strong, and smart, and funny, and handsome, and good with kids, and the best dad ever.

I looked up at him and said, "I want you. I want to hire YOU."

He laughed, and we held on to each other, sitting with that idea.

"Let's think about it," Dan said. "It's a possibility."

Over the next few days, we wrestled with our options. We put everything on the table. Unfortunately, I couldn't quit my job to stay home with the kids. My salary was higher than Dan's, and I'd gone through too many years of education to give up my tenure-track position. We also looked at daycare (which, before, we'd ruled out because Clara developed health problems when she was in daycare the first year of her life). I called every reputable center in town. There was not a single daycare with an opening right now for one child, much less three! We considered hiring another nanny, but I couldn't stomach that. The thought of going through a seventh search, likely to end in failure again, was nauseating. I couldn't do it. We talked about Dan cutting his hours to part-time, but that still left us with no one to watch our children the other 20 hours of the week.

Finally, we talked about the possibility of Dan quitting his job to be a stay-at-home parent. He'd lose his salary—it would be a big pay cut for us—but with the money we'd save from not paying for childcare, we'd just barely be able to pay our basic monthly bills. We wouldn't have any money left over for leisure activities or eating out, but our kids would benefit immensely from having a stable caregiver—a parent who loved them unconditionally and wouldn't quit abruptly or call in sick—with them every day. A bonus was that I'd have more time to work on the blog, because I wouldn't constantly be stressing about childcare.

The next day, Dan gave his two weeks' notice. He left his good-paying job to support me, to make the kids his priority, and to help out EBB. He left his friends, his coworkers, a job he loved, retirement and health benefits, and his career. And he didn't hesitate, either. He never once looked back. He announced to our family and friends that he was quitting so that he could "party with Clara, Henry, and Susie full time."

Dan's first week home, we realized that all this time we'd been trying to run a rat race, with both of us working 40–50 hours per week and hiring out childcare. Mornings and evenings and even weekends had been *so* stressful. Now, I could leave for work knowing the kids were in good hands, and that when I came home, supper would already be started. Our pace slowed. There was no doubt—with Dan at home, we were all happier and less stressed.

It also became easier for me to travel for my faculty job or to birth conferences, knowing Dan was at home. Within a few weeks after Dan quit his job, I was on a plane headed to Kansas City, Missouri for a doula conference. I'd actually taken vacation time from work so I could give a presentation at this conference, since childbirth research wasn't part of my official faculty role.

After the plane landed, I grabbed a taxi to head downtown. I was excited and nervous—what would this kind of event be like?

I walked around the conference grounds curiously. Everywhere I looked, there were doulas, doulas, and more doulas! There were vendor exhibits for rebozos (soft, handwoven scarves made in Mexico that are used for comfort during labor), MamAmor birthing dolls (handmade dolls used to demonstrate birth to children), and a booth for Spinning Babies® (a website for pregnant parents wanting resources and self-care activities to avoid Cesareans or childbirth challenges relating to baby's position in the womb).

After snatching a water bottle, I followed the crowds into the main ballroom and grabbed a seat.

An obstetrician was the keynote speaker that morning. She was speaking on "Preventing the First Cesarean," a review of factors that contribute to preventable Cesarean births. I reached for a pen and pad lying on the table and began to take notes furiously, determined to capture as much information as I could.

There were some statements the speaker made that I agreed with, like, "You can't sacrifice someone's normal vaginal delivery just because you need the room" (talking about how so many doctors will send someone to the operating room for a Cesarean because they've got other patients coming through) and "We're facing a national crisis" (in reference to Cesarean rates).

However, as she spoke, I grew disturbed by some of the phrases I heard emerging:

"How we *manage* pregnancy."

"How we *manage* labor."

"We might *let them* have a longer labor induction."

I was saddened that this obstetrician, as progressive as she was, still did not seem to understand the bigger picture. She was entrenched in the mindset that labor was something to be "managed" by obstetricians, that babies were "delivered" by doctors.

"Why," I thought to myself, "Why do so many people think they can control a bodily process?"

As the speaker came to the end of her talk, the moderator asked for questions. A group of people began lining up at the microphone. I don't know why, but I stood up and walked to the back of the line. And then, when the microphone was mine, I realized I had no idea what I was going to say.

But in the end, it didn't really matter.

I leaned toward the microphone and said, "Hi, my name is Rebecca Dekker, and I'm a nurse with my PhD, and the founder of Evidence Based Birth."

It seemed like every single person's head snapped around. There were hundreds of eyes staring at me. People were whispering and pointing. "That's Rebecca? That's Rebecca Dekker!"

I made a comment that critiqued one of the studies she mentioned and sat back down.

Eyes continued to follow me back to my seat. As I left the banquet room, I was approached by dozens of curious strangers.

"Hi Rebecca, it's so nice to meet you!"

"I am such a huge fan of your work . . ."

"I can't believe I'm meeting you in person!"

For the rest of the conference, everywhere I went, people stopped to speak with me. It was clear that the work that I was doing, this little side project, had become a really big deal. Doulas and childbirth educators from all over the world were using my website, and telling all of their friends and clients to use it, as well!

The last day of the conference, after a long day of enjoying other people's educational sessions, as well as teaching one of my own, I walked back into the ballroom for a keynote speech by Ngozi Tibbs, called "Diversity in Childbirth Education and Breastfeeding." I was interested in the topic, but didn't think I had that much to learn. We'd covered a lot of information about diversity in health care in my nursing program.

Ngozi began her session by flashing a series of photos on the screen. She asked us to think, to ourselves, what was the first word that popped into our heads when we saw each photo?

A Hispanic woman holding a baby.

"Spanish speaking," I automatically thought.

A Black pregnant woman.

"Single mom."

A plus-size woman.

"Overeating."

A person in a wheelchair.

"Disabled."

I sat there, horrified at the words that were popping into my brain. I, who prided myself on using my little bit of Spanish to establish rapport with my patients, who valued my relationships with my Black and plus-size friends and coworkers. I even have an older sister who is in a wheelchair, and she means the world to me. Yet, when I saw that picture, all I could think of was the word "disabled"?

What was wrong with me?

It turns out that what I suffered from, and what everyone possesses, is something called implicit bias.

Implicit bias is defined as unconsciously labeling members of a group as having specific qualities. This tendency—to hold unintentional stereotypes—probably stems from a basic human instinct to "categorize" groups in order to make snap judgments about potential threats. If you were a hunter-gatherer out in the wild more than 20,000 years ago, you would need to be able to quickly size up someone and the level of danger they presented.[127]

Unfortunately, today, these implicit biases permeate society. We are all raised to believe certain things about certain groups, and those beliefs seep into our subconscious. What's more, these biases lead to substantially worse health care for people from stigmatized groups. As a nurse, even if I consciously reject negative biases, as long as they exist in my subconscious, my implicit biases will affect how I understand, act, and make decisions about providing health care to people from different groups.

I sat there pondering my childhood, and asked myself: What could have led to my categorizing a Black woman in a photograph as a single mom? The answer came quickly.

I grew up in Memphis, Tennessee. Or, more accurately, I should say I grew up outside of Memphis. When I was growing up, Black people made up 63% of the population inside the city limits of Memphis. Meanwhile, in the suburb of Germantown, Tennessee, where I lived as a child, Black people were only about 10% of the population. Despite the proximity between Memphis and Germantown, I grew up without a single Black friend or acquaintance. Memphis suffered from rampant poverty and crime, while Germantown—affluent, with large brick homes on oak-lined streets—was considered the "safe" place to live.

I was raised in a home where we were taught that everybody was our neighbor, no matter who they were, where they lived, or what the color of their skin was. But I remember my friends' parents talking about Black people with a scathing tone. I remember the few Black kids in my school sitting at a cafeteria table by themselves. I remember overhearing conversations where adults said things like, "Did you hear? That neighborhood is going downhill [translation: a Black family just moved in]. The Joneses are putting their house up for sale to get out before things get worse." (What they were promoting was white flight, defined as White people moving away from neighborhoods when Black families move in.)

What I witnessed as a young child was the result of hundreds of years of racism, prejudice, and power-wielding of

White people over Black people—beliefs not only held by individuals, but written into law and policy for generations. These beliefs and structures, I later learned, were particularly powerful in former slave-holding states like the one I grew up in. As a child, I was aware of the language and actions of racism and prejudice around me, but I didn't understand what was going on, nor why it persisted. It certainly wasn't explained to me in school. Not even in college or graduate school.

Now I realized, sitting in that conference ballroom, that even though I'd consciously rejected the phenomenon of racism, and viewed it as wrong, it was still being perpetuated through me, via the simple act of my continuing to subconsciously believe harmful stereotypes.

Ngozi went on.

She began to read a poem she had written about what it's like to be a Black mom at the playground. In the poem, her child is carefree, swinging on the swing set. Another mom notices the Black child and makes a sour face. She hushes her child away while the Black mom prays her own child doesn't notice—that her child will be innocent of the effects of racism for just a little bit longer. "Swing away," she says sadly.

I was stunned. I had never before thought of innocent children being subjected to racist thoughts and behaviors. Or what it would be like to be a mom on the playground, watching other parents making ugly faces at my child, just because of the color of my baby's skin.

As I left the conference, I vowed to do as much as I could to educate myself about the effects of racism on birthing families.

What I found shocked me. According to the Centers for Disease Control, non-Hispanic Black women and American

Indian/Alaskan Native women are three to four times more likely to die during or after pregnancy and childbirth than White women. More specifically, there are 43 maternal deaths per 100,000 live births for Black women, 33 deaths per 100,000 live births for American Indian and Alaskan Native women, and 13 deaths per 100,000 live births for White women and 11 deaths per 100,000 live births for Hispanic women.[128] Nearly two-thirds of these deaths (60%) are considered preventable![129]

But it's not just maternal mortality rates that are higher. Black families are substantially more likely to experience a pre-term birth, have a low birth weight infant, lose a baby in stillbirth, and experience the death of their infant in the first year of life. What's more, researchers have consistently found that these differences between Black and White birth outcomes persist even after controlling for other risk factors, such as income level, prenatal care, and education level. In other words, these disparities are not due to socioeconomic status.[130]

If it's not because of socioeconomic status, then why are Black mothers and babies dying at higher rates?

Once I dove into the research, I found that negative birth outcomes are directly due to racism inflicted upon black women.[131,132] First, racial discrimination increases inflammatory markers of stress. Racism causes both acute stress from specific incidents of discrimination and chronic stress from a lifetime of exposure. It's documented in experimental studies that exposing Black people to racist material in laboratory settings causes an understandably negative cardiovascular response, with changes in heart rate and blood pressure.[133] Other researchers have found that Black mothers who give birth to very low birth weight pre-term infants are more likely to report experiencing racial discrimination during their life-time compared to Black mothers who give birth to normal weight infants at term, even after considering the mothers' age, education, and smoking status.[134]

What's more, it's thought that these stressors have accumu-lated over generations—an effect called intergenerational trau-ma.[135] Researchers are starting to look to *epigenetics* to explain how an environmental exposure (such as a traumatic event) can lead to a change in the function of an individual's DNA that can then be passed on to future generations. Epigenetics is a relatively new subfield of genetics concerned with how expo-sures in the environment can change our genes by switching them on and off (for better or for worse). This makes sense when you think about it. For example, when my grandmother was pregnant with my mom, the environment that shaped my grandma's pregnancy might have had an impact on the health of both my mom's and my pregnancies. That's because my mom was present as a fetus, and I was partially present as an egg, while my grandmother was pregnant! Thus, it's thought that the historical context of how women are treated during pregnancy and birth—even if it happened many years ago—can have an impact on birth outcomes today.

However, unlike my grandmother, who was White, a Black woman's grandmother would have experienced racism throughout her entire life. And so would her daughter, and her daughter's daughter. Researchers have found that babies of African immigrant mothers have outcomes more like White babies rather than U.S.-born African American babies— they are bigger and less likely to be premature.[136] But, decades later, the grandchildren of African immigrant women are more likely to be premature, like African American babies.[137] Grandchildren of White immigrants, on the other hand, are even bigger than their mothers were at birth! This is evidence that the increased risk of low birth weight and prematurity among Black babies is *not* a risk that's inherent to having Black skin or African ancestry. Instead, it's the harmful environmental exposure of racism directed towards people with brown or black skin that causes poor outcomes. In other words, these risks are not related to race. They're related to *racism*.

Before I go any further, it's important to mention that there is a common misconception that we can be categorized into different human "races." But biologically and genetically, all human beings are *Homo sapiens*—there is more genetic variability among people of a certain "racial" group than there is *between* "races."[138] The dominant viewpoint among scientists and anthropologists today is that race is a socially constructed concept used by White people to categorize and oppress people of other groups, particularly Black people.[139] This is why being "color blind" doesn't work. A White person may pretend not to notice someone's skin color, but it's unethical for the White person to ignore that society has constructed an entire system to oppress Black and Brown people, and that the White person is perpetuating that system and benefiting from it!

Second, I know there's a lot of confusion about the loaded term of "racism," so let me help clear the air. Dr. Beverly Daniel Tatum, a clinical psychologist and author of the book *Why Are All the Black Kids Sitting Together in the Cafeteria?*, defines racism as a "system of advantage based on race, that involves cultural messages, institutional policies and practices, and the beliefs and actions of individuals."[140]

Racism is often confused with prejudice. But racism, also known as white supremacy, is a system we all live in, that includes prejudiced beliefs as one part of that system. Racism is driven by the power that White people have (whether they realize it or not) to oppress others in all areas of their lives—through laws, policies, educational systems, reproduction, health, and media. On the other hand, prejudice is defined as a preconceived notion or opinion that can often lead to racist actions that perpetuate the system of racism.

Racial prejudice is likely a contributing factor to those disparately high mortality rates I mentioned earlier. That's because health care professionals don't always listen to Black women—frequently dismissing their symptoms and concerns. Now this "not listening" may not be intentional—in many cases it may be due to subconscious biases—but research has shown that it definitely happens more frequently to Black women.[141,142] A large national survey recently found that Black women, Hispanic women, Indigenous women, and Asian women in the maternity care system were twice as likely as White women to report that a health care provider ignored them, refused to answer their request for help, or failed to respond to their request for help in a reasonable amount of time.[142] Women of color were also more likely than White women to report that their physical privacy was violated and that they were shouted at, scolded, threatened, or physically abused by health care providers.

For example, a Hispanic woman in the study who gave birth in a "birth center" inside of a hospital in North Carolina described her mistreatment:

"I hated being shouted at and lied to by the midwife . . . I never dreamed that a woman would treat a laboring woman that way. She was abusive and downright mean. I was refused food and water for 26 hours. I wasn't allowed to move out of bed to walk around. I felt like I lost my autonomy over my own body. I had given up and I remember weeping when my son was born. I was at least glad he was safe. I felt like a child and I felt so unlike my usual self. These professionals broke my spirit."[142]

Years after I attended Ngozi's presentation at the doula conference, I was struck by the news reports detailing Serena Williams's complications after childbirth. In interviews, Serena describes how she realized she was experiencing a blood clot in her lungs. She had a history of blood clots and had to stop taking her anti-clotting medication because she'd had a Cesarean. The day after she gave birth by Cesarean, Serena stepped into the hallway, gasping, to alert a nurse that she needed a CT scan and IV heparin for a pulmonary embolism. The nurse thought Serena was confused from pain medications. Serena insisted they carry out a CT scan of her *lungs*, but instead, a doctor performed an ultrasound on her *legs*. Finally, the hospital staff sent her for a CT scan of her lungs, and sure enough, there were several small blood clots in her lungs.[143] If a world-class athlete like Serena Williams, who probably knows her body better than anyone, can't be believed when she's experiencing a life-threatening childbirth complication, what are the chances that other Black women will be ignored or dismissed when they speak up about their symptoms?

Now that my eyes were opened to what racism really is (a combination of oppressive systems and individual prejudices), and how it affects families of color, I've realized racism isn't just present in labor and delivery—it's everywhere in our society. Black people experience racism in many everyday settings—schools, neighborhoods, playgrounds, shopping malls, and grocery stores. Can you imagine being followed around by a suspicious store clerk while you're browsing for new clothes? Being rejected for a job interview or mortgage application because you have a black-sounding first name? Hearing that another, unarmed man in your community was killed by a police officer? These are common occurrences for people with brown or black skin.

Also, because of the way our systems are set up—including health care and housing and school systems—and because of the individual prejudice they face, most Black people are forced to think about their race on a daily basis. They also have to consciously prepare and protect their children from experiences of racism and prejudice. This constant trauma of needing to protect yourself and your children can lead to physical symptoms such as nausea, headaches, stomach aches, and anxiety.[144] It can also translate into worse birth outcomes down through the generations.

This all made sense to me on an academic level, but the day after I came home from my first birth conference, I saw the effects of racism play out in real life.

I was heading to work the next morning when a notification popped up on my phone. I'd just gotten an email, and the first line said, "Someone suggested I reach out to you about my birth experience . . ."

Once I got to my desk, I sat down and digested the information in the email. Chaundrise* was a well-educated Black woman in her early thirties who lived in a town just down the highway from me. After reading some of the blog articles on the Evidence Based Birth® website, she'd decided to switch to a nurse-midwife practice that was supportive of a wide range of birth plan options.

Chaundrise did everything she was supposed to in order to stack the odds in favor of a healthy birth. She followed all of her care provider's advice. She ate healthy foods during pregnancy, exercised regularly, went to all her prenatal visits, and went to prenatal yoga classes weekly. Her husband was supportive and attended a comprehensive six-week childbirth class with her. They felt about as prepared as they could for the birth of their first child.

Leading up to the birth, Chaundrise's plans were flexible. She expected to be able to use non-drug pain management strategies, like the hospital tub, and mobility and position changes. She thought she'd hold off on an epidural as long as possible, but she wasn't opposed to getting one if she felt like she needed it. She was looking forward to the hospital's celebratory "post-birth" meal, and the complementary massage they offered to all women who birthed there. But mostly, she hoped to be supported in this exciting and scary time of her life. Although none of Chaundrise's midwives were Black like her (she would have preferred a midwife from a similar background, but there were no Black midwives in the entire

---

* For privacy reasons, Chaundrise's name is a pseudonym, and her story is a compilation of multiple stories told to me over the years by Black families.

region—only one in the whole state, in fact), she felt good about the practice she'd chosen.

Chaundrise's water broke at 40 weeks and she headed to the hospital with her husband, with contractions immediately picking up and coming every four minutes. She arrived at the hospital, visibly in active labor.

"I need you to get in the bed so I can do a vaginal exam," the nurse directed, without even introducing herself.

"I can't!" Chaundrise exclaimed. "I can't lie on my back. It hurts too much!"

Frowning, the nurse walked out of the room, leaving Chaundrise and her husband alone. She came back in about 15 minutes later, rolling the computer on wheels for the intake exam, still with an unfriendly attitude. Chaundrise began to have a bad gut feeling about the whole situation.

As the nurse asked the long list of questions about Chaundrise's health history, Chaundrise became increasingly uncomfortable. The contractions were coming every four minutes, lasting more than a minute, and nobody had offered her any pain medication or comfort measures yet. There didn't seem to be a tub in her room, even though she'd asked for the room with the tub. Chaundrise became more anxious and fearful, and soon the pain during each contraction became unbearable.

"I think I need an epidural," she gasped to the nurse, who was still working on the intake computer form.

"You're going to have to wait," the nurse said, staring at the computer. "We have to get you checked in first."

"But can't you call the anesthesiologist?" Chaundrise's husband asked.

"I can," the nurse replied. "But it won't make any difference. Besides, it doesn't seem like the pain is that bad. She can't be that far along."

Chaundrise began moaning and swaying on the side of the bed, deep in the throes of another contraction.

"I need you to get in the bed *now*," the nurse said again, ignoring the fact that Chaundrise was in the middle of a contraction. "I have to do your vaginal exam before you can be admitted."

Chaundrise moaned and looked up, breaking her concentration. "But I don't want you to do it," Chaundrise said, gasping, "I want my midwife. She said she would do all my exams. I talked with her about that. It's on my birth plan."

"I told you," the nurse said. "I need to do your exam *NOW*. Now get in the bed if you want that epidural!"

Chaundrise got into the bed, frightened. The nurse put on gloves, then moved Chaundrise's legs apart, and began to do a vaginal exam. Chaundrise cried out in pain and said, "Stop!"

"Is that really necessary?" her husband asked.

The nurse ignored them both and proceeded to do a very rough exam as Chaundrise begged her to stop and tried to move away.

After the nurse finished, she took off her gloves and washed her hands without speaking. She then set a urine sample container on the bedside table.

"I need you to do this before I can call for your epidural," the nurse said.

"What's that?" Chaundrise asked.

"It's a urine test. It's standard."

"But I just had a urine test yesterday at my midwife's office and it was fine. What are you testing for?"

The nurse frowned, and said, "We just want to keep your baby safe. It's a drug screening test. Make sure you wipe yourself off before you fill up the cup," and walked out the door.

Chaundrise was in shock—scared and anxious. An hour later, her midwife arrived, and the midwife helped her get an epidural quickly and arranged for a different nurse to take the other nurse's place. Half an hour after getting her epidural, Chaundrise's baby was born healthy and without complications. Afterward, though, she was afraid to send her baby to the nursery for routine tests. If this was how a nurse would treat a Black woman, how rough might they be with a Black baby—with no one around to see?

After she was discharged, the anxiety wore off, and Chaundrise became furious. Later, she debriefed the entire experience with her midwife. The midwife apologized profusely for the first nurse's behavior, and admitted that how the nurse had treated her was probably related to racism.

This is what happened: the nurse, either consciously or subconsciously, saw Chaundrise as less worthy of compassion than a White patient, which affected how she behaved toward her.

First, the nurse dismissed Chaundrise's pain and withheld pain medications. A common prejudice against Black people is that they don't "feel pain" like White people. This prejudice goes back as far in time as Dr. J. Marion Sims, considered by many to be the "father of gynecology," who performed experimental surgeries on enslaved women without anesthesia, under the racist opinion that Black women don't feel pain like White women.[145]

Second, the nurse performed a non-consented, intentionally rough vaginal exam. This was obstetric violence. Imagine how much more horrifying this would have been if Chaundrise had been a survivor of rape, like 21% of American women?[146]

And third, the nurse attempted to carry out unnecessary drug testing without getting Chaundrise's consent first. This action was not only illegal (the Supreme Court ruled in 2001 that it is a violation of a pregnant woman's Fourth Amendment right for a hospital to conduct a drug test without consent),[147] but done in a discriminatory way. Like most women, Chaundrise had already undergone routine drug testing earlier in pregnancy, and the results were clearly documented in her chart—all negative. This nurse suspected Chaundrise of being on drugs only because of the color of her skin.

I wrote back to Chaundrise, expressing sympathy and anger at what she had been through. I gave her several suggestions—first, to write out her story and complaint in great detail, and second, to send it to the nurse manager at that hospital, whose email address I gave to her. I offered to help her in any way I could with the complaint process.

Chaundrise wrote back, saying that she felt discouraged by the thought that nothing might ever change. She wasn't sure if she wanted to relive the trauma by writing down her story in detail and sending it to the hospital. I encouraged her to seek out a therapist and offered to support her in any way I could.

Chaundrise did contact the hospital and, after some time, they told her that after a review, they had decided her care was "medically appropriate." They were "sorry they did not meet her expectations"—implying that her expectations, rather than their racist actions, were to blame for her dissatisfaction. She called them to say that she had never even gotten the chance to share her full story with them before they reviewed her case, and that she'd like to do so now. But they said there was no need, because the investigation was closed.

Chapter Nine

TRAPPED

A YEAR AFTER THIS ENCOUNTER, Cristen and I were hanging out on my back porch. Susie was running around outside, chasing chickens. Now that Dan was a stay-at-home parent, he'd had enough time to build us a chicken coop, and we'd been enjoying raising a backyard flock.

"It seems like she really just fits in with your family," Cristen mentioned, watching Susie. "Like she's been here all this time."

I nodded. It was true. It was hard to imagine life without Susie. She was one and a half now—with rosy cheeks and a big smile, and she absolutely loved cuddling. "Mommy, will you cuddle with me?" was a question that she asked me at least four or five times per day.

We gazed out the porch windows at our two Henrys, both three years old, who were covered in mud. They were digging a giant hole in my vegetable garden, using toy bulldozers. As we watched, one Henry stood up and ran to get the "car"—a used PowerWheels kids' car that Dan had picked up at a yard sale. The other Henry ran after him and hopped in the passenger seat. Now they were zooming around the yard, driving in circles.

It was the summer of 2015, and I had taken three weeks of vacation from work so that I could work on articles for EBB. I also took advantage of one week of that vacation time to travel to speak at a nurse-midwifery conference. I had been getting so many requests to travel and speak now! But I turned almost all of these requests down, because I hated leaving my family and I was working full time. That summer, I'd had an idea: "Since I can't travel, maybe I can teach others how to teach my classes for me?"

I asked a few of my audience members, and they said, "*Yes. Count us in!*"

So, while I was at the nurse-midwifery conference, I put out a call for applications for my new program. I decided to call it the "Evidence Based Birth® Instructor Program." I received applications from all over the U.S. and Canada. I ended up accepting eleven doulas and childbirth educators into a pilot group.

It had now been a month since I'd started the pilot, and I was impressed by these professionals—they were passionate and intelligent. It was going to be exciting to watch them spread evidence based information through the workshops they taught in their communities.

As much as I wished I could have focused all of my time on EBB and this new Instructor program, my day job at the university still took up the bulk of my time. My normal 8-to-5 workdays were filled with meetings, working on cardiovascular research trials, managing the staff on our research team, and emails, emails, emails. It seemed like I was always drowning in work emails. And now, the semester was about to start. Next week, I'd be heading to an all-day faculty "retreat," which is another word for an eight-hour meeting—how faculty traditionally celebrate the beginning of another frenetic school year.

Cristen's phone rang. "Oh sorry, I've got to get this," she said. "It's Caroline."

Cristen stepped outside to chat with Caroline. My mind drifted to Cristen's crazy life. Right now, three years after we'd met, Cristen was still doing full-time volunteer work running a national organization. Her cell phone functioned as a sort of non-funded "hotline," with Cristen as the point person for a team made up of her and a couple of dedicated lawyers. Expecting parents and doulas called and texted her day and night, reaching out for help in precarious birth and pregnancy situations, when someone's human and legal rights were being threatened or had been violated. A single parent raising her son, Cristen had quickly burned through her savings from her former life as a political and media consultant, then she'd started taking early withdrawals from her retirement savings. She'd been living below the poverty line the whole time I'd known her.

By this point, Cristen had not only used up almost all of her retirement, but she was burning the candle at both ends. She was taking care of her son by day and working all night, getting skinnier each month, and having a hard time paying rent and buying staples like toilet paper and food. And yet, like me, she couldn't stop her efforts. Even though she could have quit advocacy work and taken a well-paying full-time job in her old field, she didn't. She kept traveling around the country, sometimes at her own expense, teaching about human rights in childbirth. I paid Cristen regularly for some editing services for my blog (she is an amazingly skilled writer) and Dan and I also bartered with her so she could buy our old car, a 14-year-old Toyota. I encouraged her to start her own business, and Cristen did start a blog called Birth Monopoly. But Birth Monopoly wasn't bringing in any substantial income.

Every time I saw Cristen—whether it was at preschool where we both picked up our Henrys, or hanging out at her place or mine—she was on a phone call with someone about human and legal rights in childbirth. Recently, the someone she was most frequently talking to was Caroline Malatesta, a mother in Alabama.

A 32-year-old mother of three, Caroline had decided she wanted a different birth experience the fourth time around. The first three times, she'd had epidurals, given birth on her back, and had routine episiotomies. This time, she wanted to give birth in an upright position, use natural pain management techniques, and avoid an episiotomy. But when she asked her doctor about her birth plan, he said that was not possible at the hospital where he practiced. So, halfway through her pregnancy, Caroline switched doctors to one who said he was happy to support her birth plan—that everything she was asking for was normal practice at his hospital and healthier for her and her baby.

The hospital where this doctor worked, in fact, had been heavily marketing their support of natural or unmedicated birth. Specifically, the hospital's website and marketing materials offered women "autonomy," beautiful birthing suites with birthing tubs, "specially trained" nurses, and support for a "personalized birth plan."

But when Caroline arrived at the hospital in active labor, none of these options materialized. Her doctor was not on call. She was placed in a room without a tub, and the nurse ordered her to get in bed, on her back, so that Caroline could be placed on a continuous electronic fetal monitor, instead of the wireless monitor Caroline had requested. Nobody seemed to know or care anything about Caroline's birth plan, including her specific request (and recommendation by her doctor) to have freedom of movement.

Caroline kept questioning why she was being kept on her back, but the nurse ignored her and demanded that Caroline obey her orders. At this point, Caroline was in the midst of heavy labor, without an epidural. The contractions had gotten intense. Instinctively, she got off her back and turned over into a hands-and-knees position on the bed, which was much more comfortable for her. Her water broke, and the baby started crowning.

That's when everything fell apart.

Ordering her to her back, Caroline's nurse grabbed one of her wrists and pulled it out from under her, forcing Caroline to turn to her side so that she would not fall on her belly, while another nurse joined in the effort to put Caroline on her back. Caroline later wrote, "I desperately tried to flip back to my hands and knees, struggling against the nurses to do so. The nurses held me down and pressed my baby's head into my vagina to delay delivery as he was trying to come out."

The nurse held baby Jack's head in for six minutes, until a doctor walked in the room. At that point, the nurse released her hands and Jack came out immediately.

As a result of the obstetric violence Caroline experienced, including the awkward position she was kept in while her baby was being held inside her, she experienced a permanent injury called pudendal neuralgia, an injury of the nerves in the genital area. For Caroline, the consequences were devastating. The nerve pain in her groin area was unrelenting and untreatable, to the point that she wanted to die. She became physically unable to care for her three older children and her newborn. Her doctors told her she could not have any more children, and she could never have sex again.

Doctor after doctor told Caroline that there was no cure—that this would be a permanent condition that had altered every aspect of her life. And yet, as she thought about what happened to her, she realized after a time that she was no longer traumatized by the fact that she was injured. She could handle the pain. What she was feeling traumatized by, and hadn't really processed, was *how she was treated during her birth*. How could it be that the nurses had violated her so?

I was curious why these nurses, who probably went into nursing with the intention of *helping* people, had carried out such harmful, physical actions against Caroline. So I reached out to Dr. Mark Leary, whose Audible course "Why You Are Who You Are" had already helped me understand the difficult personalities of hospital administrators. Dr. Leary agreed to talk with me, with the caveat that since the psychology of obstetric violence hasn't really been studied, all he can do is make educated guesses about the motivation of Caroline's nurses, based on research from other fields.

When I got on the phone with Dr. Leary, he explained that the first thing I need to ask myself is, "Where is this behavior coming from?" Is it the nurses' personalities, or is it a cultural thing at this institution—or both? After discussing Caroline's situation in detail, we agreed that the nurses' actions probably originated from a combination of cultural and social norms plus the nurses' personalities. At the hospital where Caroline gave birth, this was "the way we do things here": women must be on their backs for the delivery, and the doctor must be in the room. The nurses were determined to follow these unwritten rules. In fact, hospital culture was so ingrained in these nurses—this behavior was so normalized—that later on the nurses would testify under oath that they didn't remember Caroline's birth at all.

The next thing I wanted to figure out was the *motivation* for wrestling Caroline to her back. I understood that the nurses may have had a heightened sense of conscientiousness—they wanted to follow unwritten rules, they wanted to stick to the way things are normally done—but why would they resort to physically restraining Caroline? I mean, actually wrestling a laboring woman to her back is not something a person in their right mind would do! Would *you* ever do something like that?

Dr. Leary had a couple of thoughts. His main guess was that the nurses were primarily motivated by fear.

We conjectured what might have been going on inside the nurses' heads: "I'm going to get in trouble if the baby comes before the doctor is here! She's not in her right mind; we need to take control of the situation! If I don't get her on her back right now, something bad is going to happen!"

Dr. Leary also suggested that the nurses' values may have influenced their decision to restrain Caroline. For example, maybe the nurses valued respecting traditional authority figures, such as doctors and hospital administrators and hospital policies. And maybe they valued authoritarianism much more than they valued patient autonomy. So, in a situation where a patient wants to exert their autonomy, the nurses might think, "Oh, hell, no. I'm not letting you give birth like that."

I told Dr. Leary that I was imagining a health care worker walking around a hospital with a cloud of different witnesses floating above their head, telling them what they should or should not do, with the evidence not necessarily at the forefront of their decision-making process.

Dr. Leary agreed. "A health care provider has to address a number of constituencies implicitly any time they do anything—their own values, the patient, the patient's family, the legal office, their department head . . . and they're not consciously thinking about them, but as they're walking around, there are a lot of people pulling strings on their decisions. How are they weighing the patient's desires, versus expediency, versus safety, versus not getting into trouble?"

He went on. "About Caroline's case—if I had to guess, these cases are so fear-based. A lot of stupid stuff that we do that hurts other people is that 'I'm afraid if I don't take this course of action, something bad will happen to me or them.' It's a misjudgment. It helps a little bit if you understand that some of this is well-meaning, but completely horribly executed."

Another problem that struck me about this case was how trauma goes on and on in a cyclical nature. Caroline had a traumatic birth because the nurses traumatized her, and part of why the nurses traumatized Caroline might be because they had been previously traumatized themselves!

Most people don't realize that you can develop PTSD from something that didn't happen to you directly. Instead, you can be a witness to the event and be traumatized indirectly—this is called secondary traumatic stress. Dr. Beck, whose work I described in Chapter One about birth trauma, is also an expert on secondary birth trauma. In one study with 464 labor and delivery nurses, Dr. Beck found that 35% reported moderate-to-severe levels of secondary traumatic stress, and 26% met the criteria for PTSD. That's one in four nurses, at any point in time on a hospital labor and delivery unit, who currently has PTSD![148]

It doesn't surprise me that rates of PTSD are so high among labor and delivery nurses. These nurses are there at the beginning of life, but they also intimately care for families experiencing death—stillbirths, infant deaths, maternal deaths. Back when I was in nursing school myself, I "ruled out" L&D nursing as a career because the nurses had told me too many tragic stories, and I felt I couldn't handle working there, emotionally. The nurses told me about caring for a twelve-year-old when she gave birth to an infant conceived from rape, about watching a newborn being removed from an incarcerated woman's custody immediately after birth, and being there during obstetric emergencies and "near misses" when patients nearly died from postpartum hemorrhage or other complications.

Secondary trauma is so common in birth, in fact, that Krysta Dancy, who happens to be an Evidence Based Birth® Instructor, licensed therapist, and doula, has made a career out of counseling doulas and nurses (among others) who are suffering from secondary trauma. I asked Krysta about Caroline's case to get her thoughts as well. She told me she definitely sees a link between clinicians who have secondary trauma and the perpetuation of obstetric violence with other clients in the future. "A traumatic experience is stored differently in the mind and body," she explained, "and in some stressful situations in labor and delivery, providers react to the memory of past trauma, not to the real-life situation playing out in front of them. They're suddenly dissociating."

In other words, if a health care worker is triggered by something that reminds them of a past traumatic event, they sometimes respond by detaching themselves from reality (i.e., dissociating), usually without even realizing what's happening. Their prior trauma can then take over and drive fear-based actions with the current client, even if there is no true threat at present.

Krysta also told me that she frequently sees co-dependency traits among nurses. This means that some nurses may feel responsible for another person's emotions and decisions. For example, a labor nurse might think, "I'm responsible for my patient's choices and outcomes; I might lose my license if the patient refuses to follow hospital policy." This story—that you can lose your nursing license for a patient's choice—is simply not true. But it is a story that I have heard many L&D nurses telling themselves and telling others.

The problem is, this story shifts the boundaries, so nurses think they can override the patient's autonomy. A nurse might think, "This is my room, my space, and my show; I want and know what's best for you and your baby; therefore, I must take control of the situation and you must do as I say." Sadly, many staff, who have been traumatized themselves, have no idea how they might be viewed in a client's traumatic birth story—as the *perpetrator* of trauma. They don't see that they did anything wrong, because they did everything with good intentions. And thus, the cycle of trauma continues.

Eventually, Caroline's story, and the violence she experienced at the hands of nurses (whether well-intentioned or not), ended up intertwining with Cristen's story in a big way. Two years after Caroline's injury, Cristen and Caroline met at a retreat for people working on human rights issues in birth. Cristen already knew what happened to Caroline because a lawyer colleague had emailed her a description ahead of time.

Cristen later admitted her first reaction to Caroline's story was, "Well, big deal. That shit happens to people all the time."

Her reaction wasn't surprising to me. At the time, Cristen was really worn down and experiencing a lot of secondary trauma from helping so many victims of obstetric violence. She was also showing signs of compassion fatigue. Compassion fatigue is a problem that is related to—but distinct from—secondary trauma. With compassion fatigue, Cristen had begun to lose the ability to empathize with individual women's stories—they all blurred together into this great big unsolvable problem.[149]

However, despite Cristen's secondary trauma, something in Caroline's personality—she was so authentic and selfless and persistent—resonated with Cristen. After the retreat, the two stayed in constant communication. Cristen learned that Caroline's hospital repeatedly refused to acknowledge doing anything wrong, and had declined to apologize. Caroline and Cristen began hearing from other women that they had experienced similar situations at the same hospital—being forced to give birth on their backs and being lied to about the birth options that were truly available.

Nothing was changing, and the hospital wouldn't admit any wrongdoing.

The final indignity was when a hospital administrator hung up the phone on Caroline after explaining that the hospital would not meet with her to talk about what had happened. In that moment, Caroline decided a lawsuit was the only thing they would respond to.

One of Caroline's friends from high school, Rip Andrews, was a rising star lawyer who now lived just ten minutes away. As it turned out, Rip's own children had been born near the same time, and he'd gotten a glimpse of the kind of aggression Caroline had faced when he had to advocate for his own wife during her births. Rip agreed to help her take them to court.

Unlike most people, Caroline didn't really need the money from a lawsuit. From the very beginning, her number one priority was to make sure this didn't happen to another woman at that hospital, ever again. She also knew this was her only opportunity to force the hospital to admit to what they did to her. To hold them accountable.

Now, usually, victims of obstetric violence can't find a lawyer; for the most part, if there is a healthy baby, there is no incentive for a lawyer to take the case. That's because society places very little financial value on an injured or traumatized mother. So, even if a lawyer sympathizes with a victim, it is not worth their time to bring an expensive lawsuit that won't pay off in the end. The only reasons Caroline had a chance were because a) she found a particularly creative lawyer who wholeheartedly believed in her, backed by a prestigious firm; and b) she'd suffered a lifelong injury that was clearly due to the hospital's actions, so there were actual damages that she could sue for.

On that late summer day in my backyard, with the boys zooming around in their green car, Cristen chatted on the phone with Caroline for a while, then stepped back into the back porch, holding her phone in the air.

"Guess what?" she said. "Caroline wants to use her case to help as many people as possible. We're going to get it in the news."

I knew that if anyone could get a lawsuit in the national media, it was Cristen. This was one of her specialties—getting the press to talk about hot topics. Last year, she'd traveled around the country for a new campaign called "Exposing the Silence," where she interviewed survivors of obstetric violence. Those stories had made the national news and were featured on websites like Yahoo Parenting and the Daily Mail.[150, 151] However, there was a lot of risk, for a lot of reasons, in putting Caroline's lawsuit out there in the national media. But they'd decided to go for it. Even if a jury rejected Caroline's claim and sent her home with nothing, it would all be worth it if she could get the truth about obstetric violence out to the public.

I wasn't sure that Caroline's lawsuit would be successful—most obstetric cases settle outside of court and disappear with non-disclosure agreements forbidding either party from talking about what happened. But I trusted Cristen's judgment. If she wanted to spend her time helping Caroline with her case, I knew it was the right thing to do.

The next week, my academic year started. I went to the scheduled all-day retreat feeling restless, Caroline's case weighing heavily on my mind. As I sat in the rented ballroom, along with roughly 80 other faculty and staff members from our department, I started thinking about a book Dan had recently bought me, called *First Things First* by Dr. Stephen Covey,[152] the same author who wrote *Seven Habits of Highly Effective People*.

With a start, I realized that what I was experiencing at work was a disconnect between my "clock" and my "compass."

My "clock" was made up of the demands on my time—my schedule, my work responsibilities, the classes I had to teach, the meetings I had to attend, the never-ending work emails in my inbox.

My "compass" was made up of what my inner voice was leading me to do—my vision and mission at Evidence Based Birth®, my principles and belief that every family should get evidence based care, and how I wanted to lead my life—as someone at the forefront of improving the standard of childbirth care.

Unfortunately, my compass was not present in my faculty job, and it was definitely not present in the health care institution connected with my job.

I was beginning to feel trapped.

Dr. Covey explains that there are four main needs in life—physical, social, mental, and spiritual—and that these needs are interconnected. You can't focus on your mental needs, for example, if you don't have enough money to live on to meet your physical needs. I discovered that the most synergy comes when what you do with your life fulfills all four of those needs at once.

As I was sitting there, listening to the meeting drone on, the realization struck me like a thunderbolt—I could fulfill all of those needs if I quit my job and worked solely on Evidence Based Birth®.

At the same time, I thought there was no way I could do it—the fear of leaving my job was paralyzing. And not only that, but I felt committed to my job—to my students, and coworkers, and mentors. My research mentors, in particular, had invested so much time and money into growing me as a faculty member. I loved my university and all the people I worked with. I also didn't know if it would be in my best interests to quit, since being a faculty member gave me the status of an "assistant professor" that I would have to give up. And there was this all-encompassing security attached to my job. Our website could not meet my physical needs, at least not yet. I literally couldn't afford to quit. Dan was no longer working. We wouldn't be able to get health insurance. What would we do, live off air?

It began to physically hurt to sit there at the retreat. As I listened to conversations that I'd heard repeated over and over through many years—the same arguments, the same politics, the same controversies about our nursing curriculum—I felt frustrated by the fact that not only did meetings seem to be a sort of "dead space" where change never happened, but that I was not allowed to work on childbirth research as part of my faculty role.

My mind flitted back to several years earlier, when I had asked for a meeting to discuss switching research fields from cardiovascular science to childbirth. As I sat at a conference table with my supervisors and mentors, I explained why my research interests had shifted. They listened understandingly. However, after much discussion, they decided that it would be okay for me to pursue childbirth research, but only if it was linked directly with cardiovascular research. For example, I could conduct studies about postpartum heart failure—but not postpartum care in general. Or, I could study gestational diabetes, a cardiovascular-related condition, but not the topic of informed consent in childbirth. In other words, it was okay for the blog to be my evening "hobby" or my weekend "passion," but at the end of the day, my work assignment was to seek grant funding in cardiovascular science.

I understand why they made this recommendation: they were thinking of my best interests. I'd built up a portfolio of many years of work in cardiovascular research—winning research competitions and publishing papers. It wouldn't look good on paper if I suddenly switched to a completely different topic, two years into my journey to tenure. Still, their decision stung.

Later, as I left the all-day retreat, and walked to my car, eager to get home and see my family, I tried to focus on the bright side. The next week, I would start teaching an undergraduate class about childbirth. Our program needed an elective class that would appeal to honors students, and I had been tapped to create a semester-long, 3-credit-hour elective all about childbirth.

The class, which I named "Babies Are Not Pizzas: The Science of How Babies are Born, Not Delivered," had opened for registration the past spring and filled up immediately. I even received emails afterward from students who were disappointed they couldn't get in. I'd spent part of the summer developing a syllabus and content calendar for the class.

Then, the week after the retreat, I finally met my twenty honors students for "Babies Are Not Pizzas." I arranged the classroom so we could sit in a big rectangle and see each other's faces. One by one, the students introduced themselves, told me their major, and told me why they'd signed up for the class. It seemed like all the students were incredibly excited to be there! In terms of majors, there were some nursing students in the class, but most of the rest of the students were enrolled in majors like pre-med and pre-pharmacy. For many of them, it was their first college class focused entirely on an aspect of health care. The students told me they all had an interest in childbirth, and yet most of them seemed genuinely scared to give birth themselves. I had lined up guest speakers and assignments on topics like Cesareans, birth plans, childbirth education, racism, and home birth. The two first class periods, where we focused on evidence based care and the history of childbirth, went really well. I knew that teaching this course would be the highlight of my faculty job.

I was prepping for class the next week when my supervisor called me and asked me to stop by her office to talk. So, I walked down the hallway and stepped into her corner office.

Sitting at her conference table, we chatted about non-work-related stuff for a few minutes, and then she got to the point.

"Rebecca," she said, "I've been told that you've been making negative statements about the university healthcare system on social media."

I was stunned. And confused.

From the very beginning, I'd been extremely careful to avoid using the university's name in any context with my blog or efforts to change childbirth care. So I wasn't sure how I could have been accused of saying anything negative about them on social media.

"What do you mean?" I asked. "I don't understand."

She told me that administrators of the healthcare system had been sharing screenshots of a comment I'd made about the university on my public Facebook page.

I racked my brain—I still couldn't figure out what she was talking about.

But then, she mentioned that it had to do with the hospital's Baby-Friendly® status.

"Ah, now I remember," I thought. Nearly two years earlier, in 2013, there had been a comment thread on the EBB Facebook page. I don't remember the context of the original post, but somebody had left a comment in a thread of dozens, saying something like, "Maybe they should look for a Baby-Friendly® hospital."

I had written back something to the effect of, "That's good advice in general, but it might not always work—the only Baby-Friendly® designated hospital in my town isn't the best place for mothers to give birth."

This was an accurate statement! At the time, and even at the time of my current meeting with my supervisor, I continued to hear negative reports from parents, doulas, and nursing students about their experiences there. Although babies were now getting care that promoted breastfeeding, mothers were still being confined to bed during labor, required to be hooked up to the continuous monitor, not allowed to eat and drink, being coerced or forced to birth on their back in stirrups, and many of the other practices that I'd experienced during Clara's birth.

"Yes," I explained, "I did make a comment like that several years ago. But it was not posted using my name, I never mentioned the name of the hospital, and I did not even state the name of the town or state where I lived."

I was not brave enough to add: "And my statement was true."

She nodded understandingly and said, "Still, you can never say anything negative about the university healthcare system."

She paused, then added in an even more formal tone, "You know, you can never say anything negative about any of the other hospitals in our region, for that matter. They are our community partners, after all."

"Of course," I replied. "It was wrong of me to write that. I'll go delete that comment immediately."

I left the office, my heart racing. What had just happened?

I realized, with a start, someone had invoked the chain of command and the power hierarchy that I had worked so hard to decipher. Somebody from the hospital—I don't know who, maybe one of those original nurse administrators I met with so many years ago—knew what I was doing at EBB, finally got fed up, and reported me to the higher-ups.

I was walking down the hallway back to my office when I stopped still in my tracks. It hit me—not only was someone offended, but they seemed to have been actively *searching* for materials they could use against me to get me in trouble. That comment was buried deep in a comment thread from two years ago. It's not something you would just *stumble across*.

And I had been so careful—I had never once publicly talked about how I'd had that first traumatic birth in the university's healthcare system. Every time I mentioned my first birth story to anyone, I left out the hospital's name and even the name of the city where I lived. My silence was for several reasons. First, I loved my university, and I only felt concern and care for what happened there. Second, I didn't blame anyone in particular, and I had no desire to retaliate. The type of care I'd received at their facility was typical at the time for many hospitals. My traumatic birth with Clara was an institutional, systemic, cultural, worldwide problem—not a result of "bad nurses" or "bad doctors."

But this meeting . . . this was a wake-up call. I went to my office, packed my bag, and walked outside. While unlocking my bike from the bike rack, I called Cristen, and told her what happened.

She said, "You just can't get a break, can you?"

Just like I could see so easily that Cristen was burning out from working unpaid, she could see how I was being silenced by the institution I worked for. All this time, I had never been able to speak my full truth, for fear that somebody at my university wouldn't like what I said. And now this had happened.

"What are you going to do?" Cristen asked.

"I don't know," I said worriedly. "What do you think they'll do? Do you think they might try to censor me in the future?"

"I'd say that's a strong possibility."

As I rode my bike home from work that day, feeling the late summer sun on my skin, I realized that I was facing a huge, life-altering dilemma.

Could I ethically continue to work for an institution that not only limited women's choices in labor, but also prohibited me from using my voice to create change?

But, on the other hand, could I really leave my job? I'd spent ten years in undergraduate and graduate education to get this faculty position, and here I was, just a few years away from getting tenure, which would guarantee my job for life.

I couldn't leave my nursing students. I absolutely loved teaching and mentoring them. And I cared for my colleagues. This place had been a second "home" to me for more than a decade. Furthermore, I needed this job! We needed a salary, we needed health insurance—we had to house and feed and care for our family.

I called Cristen again when I got home from my bike commute and she asked what I was going to do.

"Nothing," I told her. "I'm not going to do anything."

The truth was, I couldn't walk away from my career. I would have to figure out a way to live with this. Maybe it would all work out, if I just kept doing EBB on the evenings and weekends, and became more careful about what I said and wrote from now on. And then, when I got tenure in a few years, I would have more freedom of speech, surely!

Over the next few weeks, as I rode my bike to and from work, and as I walked up and down flights of stairs in my college's building, I let my mind wander. Even though I had decided to stay, it didn't make my situation any less precarious. I still didn't know if or when they might try to censor me again.

One night, I woke up in a cold sweat. I'd just had a nightmare. Two, in fact. In the first nightmare, I'd been standing on my front porch, and I saw the end of the world. A huge nuclear blast was headed toward me and my family. It was orange, and glowing, and the wave was about to hit our house.

In the second nightmare, I was driving in my car and I saw another car preparing to hit me head on. In the span of a few seconds, I realized I wasn't going to live to say goodbye to Dan and my children. In my dream, I died, and my spirit rose up into the air, and I looked down at my body below in my car.

I'd never actually died in a dream before—I had always woken up before it happened. But in this dream, I actually died. It felt as if it were real.

The next morning, in broad daylight, I thought about my nightmares. What did they mean? Why had I had such graphic dreams the night before?

It suddenly struck me. My dreams meant—life is short. There is no guarantee I will have a tomorrow. I should live today as if it were my last day on earth. What decisions would I make if I knew I didn't have much time left?

When I asked myself, "Who do I want to spend more time with?" I immediately answered, "My family. Dan and the kids."

And when I asked myself about my career, "Who is my responsibility to?" The answer was, "To parents and their babies."

Not to my university.

The realization was clear as day. As long as I worked within this hierarchy, I would not be truly free to advocate for families. If I wanted to make a difference in this world—to bring change to childbirth care—I had to become my own boss. I also knew that I had an aching need to spend more time with my family. On my deathbed, I wanted to be surrounded by people who loved me, whom I had gotten to spend as much time as possible with during my lifetime.

I was currently trapped in a job that prohibited me from pursuing my life's dream, from advocating for pregnant families, and from being with my family.

The answer was clear. Nobody was going to save me. I was going to have to save myself.

The question was, how?

Chapter Ten

ESCAPE

A FEW WEEKS LATER, I was on a flight to Washington, D.C. This cardiovascular conference was the last place I wanted to be going, but I didn't have a choice. I was slated to give two different presentations—one about early career advice for new faculty, and a second presentation about postpartum heart failure.

While sitting in the very back row of the airplane, I leaned my elbows onto the tray table and put my head in my hands, musing about my situation. If I wanted to quit my job, I should leave when my contract expired, at the end of June 2016. Right now, it was September of 2015. This meant I had roughly nine months to figure out how to survive without a regular paycheck.

But I'd read the fine print in detail. If wanted to leave at the end of June, I was required to give my notice in February.

So, in reality, if I was going to make a decision by February, I only had five months.

Then, while I was lost in thought, I felt a tap on my shoulder. I turned around. The flight attendant was smiling down at me.

"I was just reading the back of your shirt," she said, "And I love it."

I was wearing a t-shirt I had designed called the "Top Five Myths about Birth, Debunked," that listed five myths about birth, along with an accurate, research-backed statement that debunked each myth. One of the myths debunked said, "Big babies are not an evidence based reason for Cesarean."

"When I was in labor," the flight attendant said, unprompted, "A doctor came in and told me that my baby was too big and that there was no way I could deliver vaginally. I was crushed. But my nurse, she was on my side. She told me he was wrong, and then she helped keep that doctor out of the room for most of my labor. When it came time to push, I did it!"

It might seem odd to you that a random stranger told me her birth story in an airplane, but to be honest, this type of interaction is a pretty common occurrence for me (especially on airplanes). I wear a lot of Evidence Based Birth® t-shirts, and people almost always come up to me and ask me about the sayings on the front or back. And even if I'm not wearing an EBB t-shirt, for some reason, when people ask me what I do, the conversation leads straight to EBB. Every single time, they share their birth story with me, and it is always emotional for them. Sometimes they relate a story that is positive and empowering, like this flight attendant, and sometimes it is traumatic and disempowering.

As the flight attendant walked away, I started thinking about how birth touches so many people's lives . . . No, wait, I corrected myself. Birth literally touches *everyone's* life, because we are all born! Surely, with this much interest in what I was doing, there had to be a way to turn my blog into something that simultaneously paid me a living wage and let me fulfill my mission in the world.

Now that I thought about the possibility of creating a sustainable business, I realized I already had a lot of the beginning pieces in place.

Website with lots of content that brings in visitors from all over the world? Check. We had more than a million visitors to the website in the past year.

Potential customers? Check. I now had about 5,000 people subscribed to my email newsletter.

A problem that people desperately want solved, and are willing to pay someone to help them solve? Check. The lack of evidence based care in childbirth care really stressed a lot of people out, including me!

However, despite these assets, I was missing something big—namely, sufficient revenue to pay my salary so that I could support my family. There definitely wasn't enough traffic to the site to make a living off of advertisements, and I didn't want to create any conflicts of interest by having paid "sponsors." In September, I'd enrolled 50 more childbirth educators and doulas in our Evidence Based Birth® Instructor Program. However, that program, although a great way to spread the word about evidence based information, definitely wouldn't cover my living expenses, as it barely paid for the digital and human resources it took to run the website. At this point I had two virtual assistants working for me, helping care for the growing number of EBB-related tasks, and I needed to pay their wages as well.

I thought about the possibility of selling more online courses. Over the past few years, I'd sold a couple of one-off courses, where people could pay about $30 to take an online continuing education course from me. But a few months after each course was released, sales would dwindle off to almost nothing. It didn't seem realistic to be able to launch and promote a new continuing education course every month or two. If I was going to support my family, I needed a source of income that was more stable and predictable.

I was sitting in my hotel room that night, mulling over this problem—how to create a sustainable business model—when I decided to listen to a podcast called the "Flipped Lifestyle Podcast."

Shane and Jocelyn Sams, the hosts of this podcast, were schoolteachers in a rural town in Kentucky. They both started websites in their spare time, which eventually allowed them to quit their teaching jobs and work entirely from home. They called it the "Flipped Lifestyle" because their lives were upside down from most people's—they didn't depend on an employer for a paycheck. Instead, they created their own.

The specific solution to my revenue problem was right there, in a recent episode. I texted Dan the link: "You HAVE to listen to this podcast."

The next day, I got dressed and ready to attend the conference. I crammed a bit, studying my presentation notes, then decided to wing the rest. Today's subject was something I'd presented on before—it would be easy. Painful, because I didn't want to be there, but easy.

The convention center was frigid, as conference rooms usually are—designed for men with male metabolisms wearing long sleeves and suits. Even in my layers topped with a wool jacket, I was shivering. It felt a bit like a funeral, with researchers slowly walking around like ghosts in dark business attire. I walked down the carpeted hallway and found the room where I was giving my first talk of the day. There were about ten people who chose to attend the Early Career Session.

"Ugh," I thought. "I flew all the way to D.C., leaving my kids behind, to give a talk to ten people?"

As I sat there, my fingers and toes freezing, I waited for the presenter who was going immediately before me to finish. I was only half listening when all of the sudden something she said caught my attention.

"Courage," she said, "is not the absence of fear. Courage is acting despite your fear."

I have no idea what the rest of her talk was about. All I knew is that those words struck a chord somewhere deep inside me. It was the encouragement I needed in that very moment. Even though I knew it was the right decision to leave my job, I had been scared to do it—was still scared to do it!—and fear had been holding me back for years now. That is what I'd been lacking—the knowledge that it's okay to be scared. It's okay to be afraid. Do what you have to do anyway.

I came home from the conference ready and determined to spend every evening working on the plan I'd developed after listening to Shane and Jocelyn's podcast. Mentally, I was ready to leave my job, and so I was able to move forward with the game plan. But emotionally, I was a wreck.

I realized I needed a mentor, or a coach, or somebody I could talk with about leaving my job. Why? Well, my whole adult life I'd relied on mentors to advance my career. There's something amazing about being able to ask someone more seasoned than you for advice—to get their honest opinion. Only problem was, who could I ask for help now? I'd never known a single person who'd left an academic job to start their own business. Could a stranger give me advice? And could I trust them to hold my conversation in complete confidence?

Through an Internet search, I found a website called "The Professor Is In" that focuses on helping professors find jobs inside and outside of academia. They offered a 30-minute consulting call, and I scheduled one immediately. Cristen also put me in touch with a friend of hers, Jodi Hume, who provides decision support and coaching for entrepreneurs and startup founders.

Time was of the essence, so I was relieved when both people were able to speak with me that very week.

Jodi spent a total of three hours on the phone with me, walking me through all my options, looking at my financial situation, analyzing my emotions, figuring out a time line for when I would have to have everything completed with my business in order to quit. She also had a calming effect on me, refocusing me on the *why this decision was right* when I couldn't stop thinking about my fears and guilt.

"Rebecca," she said, "This is the work you are meant to do in the world. You are going to make such a difference in people's lives. Don't let your anxiety hold you back from ful-filling your potential!"

The other consultant, from "The Professor Is In," helped me sort out the logistics of how to actually resign from an academic job. I also talked with her about how I was deeply concerned about what my coworkers would think; I was afraid of my boss's and mentors' reactions. She reassured me that they probably wouldn't be angry—in fact, everyone might even be a little bit jealous! I had also been feeling guilty because the university and my mentors had invested so much money and time into my education and career. She reminded me that I'd already given back by providing my university with publications, presentations, classes, and grant funding. She said that I couldn't put my entire life on hold just because they'd helped me in the past.

Their support, along with Dan's, helped me get through the next two weeks.

And then, it was time to put the plan into action. The revenue part, at least.

I sat down at my home office in the basement—the same chair where I'd been sitting when I felt that first pressure wave with Susie's birth. I took a deep breath and composed an email to the more than 5,000 people who subscribed to my newsletter.

> Subject line: Big Announcement!!
>
> I have to admit, I'm a little nervous to be sending you this email today. What I'm about to announce is a really big deal to me! But as a really wise person once told me: Courage is not the absence of fear. So,

I'm going to go ahead and tell you my news, even though I'm scared!

What's my big news?

Well, for the past year I have been dreaming up a way that Evidence Based Birth® could play a role in *getting evidence into practice.*

I definitely want to continue to publish high-quality articles and make evidence freely available to the public. That part of EBB is not going to change!

But, I also want to help people put that evidence into practice. Because as we all know, evidence by itself is useless, if it's not actually being followed!

And with an evidence-practice gap of 15 years— meaning it takes about 15 years for evidence to be used in the hospital setting . . . well, that's not acceptable to me. And I want to start actually doing something about it.

I decided that the best way for me to tackle this problem was to use three strategies:

Start bringing people together in a community, to talk about how we can put evidence into practice.

Create a course on the steps of HOW families can get evidence based care, and train professionals and parents on these steps.

Continue to offer relevant and exciting trainings to professionals in the field who are at the forefront of putting evidence into practice.

So basically, what I have proposed (and well, went ahead and created) is a *professional membership to*

Evidence Based Birth®, with all three of these aspects included!

I'm ready for those of you who want to become the very first Evidence Based Birth® Professional Members.

If you want to learn more about how you can get early access to the professional membership, click here!

I hope you have a great week, and I am excited about what the future holds for all of us!

Sincerely,

Rebecca

I sat and stared at the email I'd written, holding my breath. Then I closed my eyes, inhaled, exhaled, and clicked "Send."

I couldn't sit around and watch. It was too painful to imagine the crushing failure I'd feel when, hours from now, I would open up my email to find zero sales and a host of angry emails from people, incensed that I had the nerve to charge for my work. You have to understand that, in the birth world, there's a lot of internalized sexism. Several women I knew, who blogged about childbirth for a living, had been openly criticized—no, outright shamed—for charging for online services. The prevailing thought among many in the field was that women like me should be doing this work for free (for surely, there must be a man paying my bills!).

I closed my laptop and headed to work.

About 15 minutes before my afternoon class, curiosity got the better of me. I logged into my EBB email. Thirty-five people had already joined as Professional Members! I couldn't believe it! And the emails coming into the inbox weren't negative . . . instead, people seemed excited I was creating this opportunity.

As the week went on, my hope began to grow that maybe, just maybe, the birth community would rally around me and support my work, so that I could write about the research on childbirth full time. Within a week, the day of the registration deadline, I knew we were on to something. More than 100 people from around the world had joined the Professional Membership and had committed to paying either monthly or annually for this service, and all I had done that week was send two emails!

Dan and I were excited. We could almost sense the freedom this program could bring. During Christmas break, we set our goal. If I could get a total of 200 people inside the membership, that would create a stable, predictable revenue that paid about 75% of our bills. I could then give my notice in February, figuring that by the end of June I would be closer to 100%.

On January 19, 2016, I released a series of free videos teaching about evidence based care and explaining how people could join the Professional Membership. By the end of the next seven-day period, we had broken the 200-member mark.

Dan and I hired a babysitter so that we could get some kid-free time to figure out next steps. We drove to our favorite restaurant on a cold, snowy Sunday night, and perched on top of tall stools.

We stared at each other across the table.

"So?" I asked. "What do you think we should do?"

In less than 10 minutes, we agreed that it was time for me to turn in my notice. The benefits of working for myself were too great—think of the work I could do if I were unfettered and free! The amount of research I could put into the public's hands! And now that I had created a stable, predictable revenue, it seemed like we wouldn't have to worry month-to-month about how we would pay our bills. We wouldn't have anybody providing retirement or health insurance for us anymore, but on the other hand, the risks of staying at my faculty job appeared too great—the possibility of censure or burnout, the ethical dilemmas.

I find it ironic that in the end, we used a combination of evidence (data/numbers and info about benefits and risks), coaching from experts, and our values, goals, and preferences to make this major life decision. In other words, it was "evidence based"!

We drove home that night brimming with excitement. A whole new life was unfolding before us. A life where we could work from home together, doing nothing but raising our family and pursuing a passion to help more families get evidence based care.

There was just one barrier left.

How could I possibly get up the nerve to actually make an appointment with my dean to give her my notice? And worse, how could I possibly break the news to my mentors at the university, who depended on me as part of their research team, and had invested hundreds of thousands of dollars into my education, with the expectation that I would have a long, fruitful career as a nursing professor? I thought I'd worked through that guilt with my coaching sessions, but apparently it was still deeply bothering me.

On the first day after my date with Dan, I didn't take any action to make an appointment with my dean. On the second day I didn't, either. Then, on the third day after we'd made our decision, Clara and Henry (now ages 7 and 3) had a dental appointment at a pediatric dentistry clinic for a routine cleaning. Now I know you might be wondering, "What does the dentist have to do with this story?"

Well. Let me tell you.

My dental insurance offered several plans, and the one we had (the cheapest) only covered care at the university's own dental clinic. This clinic mostly sees children on Medicaid and those who have no insurance. They make no effort to cater to children. The entire environment is sterile, clinical, and scary looking. There are no windows, and no kid-friendly decorations. But this was the option we had.

Our kids had appointments at the same time. Dan headed off with Henry, led by a grouchy-looking hygienist, and I went with Clara, following a hygienist who looked equally as irritable. As Clara got in her chair, I heard Henry beginning to cry in fear a few booths down.

Clara was visibly nervous. She has a thing about some toothpaste flavors—she hates the texture and taste, so we'd brought her preferred toothpaste along, which I tried to hand to the hygienist, offering a little explanation. She ignored me. She never smiled at us, and she did not introduce herself.

She gestured at the chair. Clara sat down.

As the hygienist lowered the head of Clara's chair, Clara squirmed, trying to sit up. "Put your head down," the hygienist commanded. Then the dentist walked up. He was an older gentleman wearing a white lab coat.

Clara became more and more nervous. She'd never met this dentist before, and he didn't introduce himself or say anything to her. She laid her head back down, and obediently opened her mouth, but as he reached for the toothbrush, covered with the clinic toothpaste, she panicked and started crying and trying to sit up. The dentist growled at her, "Put your head back down!"

She started bawling.

I said, "Please don't do that. Please just use the toothpaste we brought along. She has sensory issues and she will not tolerate your toothpaste."

He looked at me with disgust.

Then he bent forward and put his hand back down on her shoulders, restraining her, and grabbed the toothbrush to do it anyway.

Clara was straining and shaking and sobbing, tears streaming down her face.

I said, "STOP. STOP RIGHT NOW. I do not give you permission to do that. I refuse any further care."

I grabbed my daughter and pulled her out of the chair. Clara was shaking and sobbing. The dentist and the hygienist looked at me like I was a crazy person.

My legs started shaking uncontrollably underneath me.

I said, "I would like to speak with a manager right now."

The dentist raised his voice and said furiously, "I *am* the manager. You can talk to me right here, right now."

Still shaking, I attempted to have a conversation with him and the hygienist, but it was increasingly clear that they were defensive and angry with me. Every time I tried to explain why I was upset, and what they were doing was wrong, that there are ways to help kids cope with anxiety that don't involve physical force, he shot me down and said, "Well, *we* need to keep your daughter *safe*. *That's* why we have to restrain her."

Finally, I gathered my courage and said, "You know what, I'm not going to continue this conversation any longer. I will speak with a different manager at a later time."

I took Clara by the hand, grabbed our coats, and hurried to the door. As I glanced behind, I saw that a dental student had been watching the whole encounter. She was frozen in place—pale and silent.

When I got out into the lobby, I asked the receptionist to get the real clinic manager (there was one). The manager came and found me, and we went to her office and spoke respectfully. She agreed with my concerns—that the staff were not using developmentally appropriate ways to deal with child anxiety—and told me that they would talk about these issues in their staff meeting that very day. I left feeling much calmer and glad that somebody actually cared. At the same time, I knew that I would never bring my children back there.

Dan took the kids back to school, and I made my way back to my office, which happened to be in the building next door to the dental clinic.

I sat down at my desk, feeling nauseated. I had just found out that Henry had a similar experience as Clara, and Dan had left feeling just as sick and shaky as me. Henry is normally a loving, cooperative child—everybody knows he's a total sweetheart, and he always does what his parents and teachers tell him to do. But he was nervous, as this was just his second visit to the dentist, and he was afraid to lay his head back in the chair. At one point, his particular dentist made a joke, and Henry calmed down and laughed, but then the dentist went right back to forcefully doing things to him—holding his head and shoulders down and encourage him calm down.

I had recently read *Mastering Respectful Confrontation* by Joe Weston, and I was so grateful for the techniques in that book.[153] It was this book that taught me how to use the "Stop!" method if I encounter severely aggressive behavior. That's why, when the dentist used physical force and threatened my child's emotional and physical safety, I had yelled "Stop!" However, I made one mistake. I tried to engage with the dentist when he was being highly aggressive. Weston says that when someone is threatening your safety or the safety of one of your loved ones, you cannot engage in conversation with them. You simply have to get out of the situation.

I had initially purchased Joe Weston's book with childbirth and Caroline's case in mind, focusing on how to use communication techniques when health care workers are being disrespectful in labor and delivery situations. I had no idea that similar harmful behaviors—use of force and physical restraint—were being used in a pediatric dental clinic just a couple hundred feet from my office.

Does anyone else see a parallel to birth?

In this dental clinic, my children were categorized as simply *children*—lesser beings who do not have names or autonomy and must follow the rules for the sake of tradition and "safety." If they don't follow the norms, then it is appropriate to use physicality to enforce the adult's preferences on the child. If they fight back, then the staff must retaliate to show the child who is boss. The parents are only slightly higher in status than the child; they don't have the right to question the dentist's actions. The dentist assumes he has the ultimate authority to use force on a child, without asking for parental consent.

The child is a task that must be performed. The teeth must be cleaned, with the exact instruments and method that the staff choose. In the end, the child is nothing more than a lesser being's mouth. And mouths don't have feelings, or psyche, or trauma. You can do whatever you want with a child's mouth. And all the while, students are watching.

In some labor and delivery units, people who are there to give birth are categorized simply as pregnant *patients*—lesser beings who do not have names or autonomy and must follow the rules for the sake of tradition and the "safety" of their baby. If they don't follow the rules, then it is appropriate to use coercion, pressure, lying, bullying, shaming, and occasionally even physicality to enforce the health care worker's preferences on the pregnant woman. The partner is slightly higher in status than the pregnant person, but the partner is usually uneducated and afraid to speak up. The doctor may assume that the doctor has the ultimate authority to make the patient do whatever the doctor wants, without asking for consent, or even despite explicit refusal.

The patient is a delivery that must be performed. The delivery must be performed through a birth canal (i.e., vagina or an abdominal incision), with the exact instruments and methods that the doctor chooses. In the end, the pregnant woman is nothing more than a procedure happening in a birth canal. And birth canals don't have feelings, or psyche, or pain, or trauma. You can do whatever you want to with a birth canal. You don't need to ask permission to insert your hand in the birth canal, or yell at it, or cut it. And all the while, students are watching.

From this point forward, I refused to be part of that system. It is wrong.

It is wrong to view children as lesser beings who don't have the right to compassionate, evidence based care. It is similarly wrong to see pregnant people as lesser beings who don't have the right to say "yes" or "no." This is not the kind of world I wanted to be a part of anymore.

The next morning I woke up and I wrote my letter of resignation.

I emailed it to Cristen, and she loved it. She mentioned it was funny timing, as she was working on a letter to resign from the full-time volunteer work she'd been doing. I was glad to see that she would finally strike out on her own. It was like we were both breaking free at the same moment.

The day I turned in my letter, I sat at my desk all morning, anxious, unable to focus on work. As the clock ticked closer to 11 a.m., the time of my appointment with the dean of my college, I nervously called Dan.

"I don't know if I can do this!"

"It's okay," he answered. "Just get it over with."

Have you ever gotten on a roller coaster that was too tall or too wild for you? You know, when you're on that cart, inching up the hill, heading for the top of the track, looking down at the rest of the world so tiny and small? It's a crazy feeling, like, "What the heck am I doing here and can I get off?" That's the feeling I got as I walked down the stairs to my dean's office. It felt as if I had just strapped myself into a roller coaster—a hard metal bar locked against my hips. There was no turning back, no way to escape.

The only way out was forward.

Chapter Eleven

FREEDOM

DAN AND I FLOATED down the creek in a canoe, gazing at the trees that were still green, with a hint of yellow. It was early October 2018, and it was still warm—we were comfortable in shorts and t-shirts, wearing navy blue life vests. The water level was high, but calm, with just a few ripples and mild rapids. It was Monday, and nothing was in sight except wildlife. An eagle rose up from the cliffs, flapping its wings into the sky, where it soared in the air above us.

"I can't believe we are free to do this," I said.

"I know," echoed Dan. "It's crazy, huh?"

It had been more than two years since I'd walked away from my boss and coworkers and institutional responsibilities. I had built it up in my head that the dean and everybody else in my college would be so angry with me—that they could never forgive me for walking away. I was surprised to find that people weren't mad at all. They were sad to see me go, and happy that I was following my passion to become a full-time advocate for evidence based care.

Ten years ago, I never could have predicted where I would be today. To get here, I followed my passion and my gut and a never-ending hope that I could do something, anything, to change childbirth care. And now, I was living what seemed to be a dream life, both personally and professionally.

On normal workdays, Dan and I share a home office in the former nursery. My desk sits next to a window overlooking our vegetable garden, and my chair sits in roughly the same spot where both Susie and Henry were born! During the day, I work on creating content for EBB, while Dan does all of the accounting for the website. When Susie gets home from preschool, the three of us eat lunch together, then I continue working a little longer while Dan plays with Susie. At 3 p.m., when our older kids get home, both their Mommy and Daddy are waiting to greet them with hugs and kisses and "How was your day?"

It's hard to believe, but Susie, now four, can't even remember a time when both Mommy *and* Daddy weren't home with her.

Most people interrupt me at this point to say, "Wait, did you say you share the same office?"

And I say, "Yes, our desks are right across from each other, in the same room."

"What is that like?"

"Amazing."

I know some people say they could never work with their spouse all day long, but Dan and I have been best friends for a really long time now. We love hanging out together. It's always been that way between us. So that part of my life—the fact that I get to spend all day and night with Dan—well, it's pretty joyful.

Also, I'd never thought of myself as unhealthy during my years as an assistant professor, but after leaving my job, with more time to focus on my well-being, I found a diet that successfully controlled my migraines—from 15 to 20 episodes per month down to 2 to 4. A surprising side effect of this lifestyle change was that I lost 20 pounds and was now back to the same weight and energy level I'd had on my wedding day.

One big sacrifice we made when I left my job was health insurance. We were able to buy a health insurance plan for our family for the first six months after I quit my job, in the second half of 2016. Unfortunately, after that, the cost of health plans on the Affordable Care Act exchange skyrocketed. In early 2017, we realized that monthly health insurance premiums were going to be *more expensive than a mortgage payment* and have incredibly high deductibles, leaving us to foot the bill for the first $5,000 of all medical care that year. We didn't qualify for assistance, and yet we couldn't afford the health plan on our own. So, we decided to stop purchasing traditional health insurance altogether. We signed up for a catastrophic health plan that would cover an unexpected hospitalization, but didn't cover pre-existing conditions, maternity care, immunizations, medications, laboratory testing, mental health care, or more than 2 doctor's visits! We did, however, find a direct primary care clinic that could provide us with unlimited primary care and urgent care for a monthly fee, as well as medications and laboratory tests at wholesale prices.

So we don't have regular health insurance, but on the other hand, we're free. *I'm free.*

Our lives are so flexible now. The 9-to-5 grind vanished. When I work on EBB stuff, it doesn't really feel like work, because I'm so passionate about what I do. If I need to take time off for family—to go on a field trip with Clara or Henry, or spend time with my mom or dad—I just do it, without asking anyone. Today, in honor of our 15th anniversary, Dan and I spontaneously chose to skip work and go canoeing together instead.

Who would have ever thought that I would go from being a nurse, to a graduate student, to an assistant nursing professor, to an . . . entrepreneur?

Dan and I saw a rocky beach and directed our canoe there to take a break and snap some photos. As I hopped out and helped pull the canoe to shore, I thought about how not only my daily life had changed completely, but also my perspective. I'd gone from being naïve about birth, and determined to follow hospital policy, to being a leader in the movement to help families get better, safer care in the hospital setting.

And none of this would have happened if I hadn't had that first traumatic birth with Clara.

It still makes me sad, and a little angry, that they separated us at birth for hours.

But mostly, I just feel sad.

I still get a lump in my throat whenever it's brought up. And yet, I feel fortunate that I was able to take that trauma and turn it into something positive and productive that could help other people. It was not the trauma itself that led me here, but rather my *struggle* with the aftermath of the trauma that allowed me to experience something that Dr. Cheryl Beck calls "perinatal post-traumatic growth."[154] Post-traumatic growth doesn't happen to everyone who's had a traumatic birth, but people who've experienced this phenomenon describe feeling stronger and changed forever. They empathize more with other people, form deeper relationships with family and friends, and become more assertive and more willing to use their voice to stand up for themselves and for others.

I identify a lot with the women in Dr. Beck's studies on post-traumatic growth. Because the truth is, like they said, I was broken by the system. But now, I am unbreakable.

My thoughts turned to Cristen. She was happier and less stressed now as well. That's because Cristen's hard work with Caroline had paid off in a big way. It all came to a head when Caroline's trial began in Alabama, a few weeks after my last day at the university.

Cristen stayed with Caroline the entire two weeks of the trial. She acted like a legal doula—providing Caroline with emotional support and poring over aspects of the trial with Caroline and the rest of the team each night. I was visiting family in Michigan with Dan and the kids, and every night I eagerly awaited Cristen's texts, so I could stay updated on the case.

The hospital's defense strategy was to point fingers at Caroline and blame her for the pudendal nerve injury. They argued that Caroline showed she did not care about her baby's safety when she refused to get into the "traditional" delivery position in stirrups. They painted the hospital as the savior of the baby, and Caroline as a bad, selfish mom. But Cristen could tell that the mostly female jury wasn't buying it.

The last day of the trial arrived, and Caroline finally got on the stand. There was electricity in the air as everyone waited with bated breath to hear what she would say. Caroline spoke plainly and calmly about what happened and related the extent of her injury. Her story deeply affected the jury—they passed around tissue boxes, and two of the jurors held hands, tears streaming down their faces as they listened to Caroline's story.

Then the hospital's defense lawyer began his final line of questioning. Cristen said she was incredulous as it dawned on her, but she couldn't think of any other possibility for his bizarre questions: it seemed like he might actually believe Caroline cared more about her birth experience than the life of her baby, and that she would admit to that on the stand.

> Defense attorney: "And certainly, if it were between using a wired monitor and no monitor at all, you were okay with using the wired monitor?"
>
> Caroline: "I mean, it certainly was one of the biggest reasons why I moved [from one hospital to the other], but had I come into that room and there was no wireless monitor, I did not want to go without monitoring my baby. And I could have moved around on the wired monitor, at least tried to move off my back."
>
> Defense attorney: "And certainly, if the monitor had shown something that required some emergency change of plan, such as an emergency that required a C-section . . . you were okay with that, changing your plans to respond to whatever the monitor showed?"
>
> Caroline: "I would have done anything. I mean, based on the monitor and the doctor saying it's not

looking right. I think we're sort of past that point, though, when the baby came."

Defense attorney: "At that point, though . . . well. You wanted a safe delivery, didn't you?"

Caroline: "Absolutely. That was my first priority."

The defense attorney shuffled his papers and said, "Your honor, may I have just a moment? . . . Thank you. That's all I have."

Cristen thought, "That's it. This trial is over. We've won."

After 10 hours of deliberation, the jury walked back into the courtroom and announced their verdict. They found the hospital guilty of malpractice and reckless misrepresentation of fact. They awarded Caroline $10 million in compensation for medical expenses for her permanent nerve injury, $1 million to her husband for loss of consortium, and $5 million in punitive damages for reckless fraud related to the hospital's marketing campaign promising to support "natural birth."

Not only did Caroline receive validation when the jury recognized that she was wronged, but with Cristen's help, the national media picked up the story—shining a bright spotlight on the problem of obstetric violence, and non-evidence based care during childbirth.[155,156,157]

Perhaps my favorite thing about the verdict was that Caroline chose to take a portion of the money from the verdict and donate it to create a family foundation with several years of funding. Caroline named this new foundation the "Birth Monopoly Foundation," in recognition of Cristen's hard work and sacrifice. And Cristen was hired as the foundation's sole paid employee.

Cristen was now free to pursue her advocacy goal—to bring awareness to the problem of obstetric violence. She began working on a documentary with Caroline, called "Mother May I," all about informed consent in childbirth.[158,159] And to all our relief, Cristen wouldn't have to worry where she'd find money to buy groceries each week.

As Dan and I got back in the canoe and pushed off from shore, I tossed my phone to him. I needed to do a live video stream for my audience. He held the phone and filmed, while I steered the canoe and talked to our followers from all over the world. It was time to announce registration for the first large Evidence Based Birth® Conference, which I would be hosting the next year.

Working at EBB full-time was a lot of fun. This inter-professional conference, which had always been a dream of mine to host, ended up selling out a whole year in advance. It was strange, but now that I had so much more time from quitting my job, it seemed like all the projects I touched were successful. We'd started a podcast and a new Higher Ed program for colleges and universities. And the Professional Membership, the project that created the financial stability so that I could quit my job, was thriving. We had nearly 500 members now, and the number was growing each year.

To help with the workload, we had seven contractors doing regular work for us, and we'd just hired our first full-time employee. Not only was EBB supporting our family, but it was allowing other people—most of whom were stay-at-home parents—to support their families as well. Although I had toyed with the idea of turning EBB into a non-profit, in the end I decided to keep it a company, or, what we call it, a "for purpose" company. We continually invested the money we earned back into improving the research articles and other free resources we offered to the public. Our structure was nimble, and I had hopes that we would continue to be able to effect change worldwide.

Often, when people find out I left my job, they ask me, "What's your favorite part about working at EBB full-time?" I always answer that my favorite part is working with the Evidence Based Birth® Instructors. The little pilot I started in 2015 has grown to more than 150 professionals from all over the world. Our EBB Instructors are highly experienced doulas, childbirth educators, nurses, midwives, and chiropractors who we train to teach our content. Now, we are even getting obstetricians in our program! I absolutely love watching the EBB Instructors create change using the strategies we teach them in the program—building bridges and working on culture change in hospitals. And one of the main strategies that we train our Instructors to use is love—through words of affirmation, service, gifts, and connection to hospital staff.

Remember that power activity I did in Chapter Five? Well, love is a big "ticket out" of the top-down hierarchy! Hospital staff—nurses, midwives, and physicians—they're hurting, and so many of them are so traumatized. As the saying goes, "Hurt people hurt people." My theory is, if we communicate love to people who are hurting, that might be the most powerful intervention of all. Because if we want hospital staff to make big changes to their behavior and culture, they have to feel secure first. They have to feel loved.

I wish I'd discovered this secret a long time ago—that hospital staff are resistant to change because they're hurting and in need of love. The whole time I worked for my university, nothing ever seemed to change in the labor and delivery unit. Not for eight long years after Clara's traumatic birth. Not only was my feedback rejected, but I heard that some of the nurses there really disliked what I was doing and resented my presence on campus. To give one example, about a year after I left my job, I stopped by a university party. Someone introduced me to one of the university's labor and delivery nurses. I smiled and said, "It's nice to meet you!" Realizing who I was, this nurse literally rolled her eyes, crossed her arms, and turned away, refusing to say a word to me. It still seemed kind of strange that, at my own university, my skills and research weren't wanted at their labor and delivery unit. My guess was that I was perceived as a threat to their way of doing things—a challenge or critique of their medicalized birth culture. Maybe, if I'd been given an opening, or a chance to talk with them, communicating love could have worked. Or maybe nothing would have worked back then, because their hearts just weren't ready.

I did find relief in the fact that some positive changes seemed to be hovering on the horizon! I'd heard that the university hired a group of nurse-midwives for the first time in decades. The nurse-midwives were even permitted to purchase inflatable tubs and use intermittent auscultation! However, I also knew that introducing midwives to the nurses and doctors there wouldn't be an easy transition for anyone. I worried about the midwives having their practices restricted by the physicians or being sabotaged or undermined by some of the nurses. But I also had hope that the new graduate nurses, medical students, and new residents would be inspired by the midwives' way of practicing. That the midwives' presence and demonstration of the midwife model of care (including respect for patient autonomy), would be the start of a new, more open-minded culture.

Maybe in another ten years, childbirth care will have improved so much, not only at my former university, but in so places around the world, that people who read about my birth experience with Clara will say, "I can't believe that happened to you! It sounds like you gave birth on another planet!"

But in the meantime, we're not quite there yet. Although some hospitals and providers are providing excellent care, there's still a lot of work to do.

Frustrated by the stories of local families who were struggling to get evidence based care, I decided to pilot a new Evidence Based Birth® Childbirth Class in early 2018. First, I held online focus groups with parents to see what they thought about childbirth education. I was shocked and saddened to find that most of them thought that childbirth education was a waste of time: "The only thing you learn is where to park."

They also made comments like, "My partner and I don't have time in our busy work schedules to attend classes," "Childbirth classes are awkward and embarrassing," and "I can just search online for everything I need to know." Most disturbing of all, some of them told me, "I'll just show up at the hospital and my doctor will tell me what to do."

Well, as you remember from Chapter One, that plan didn't work out well for me.

But what can I possibly do to change their minds? To convince them to educate themselves at least a little bit?

So, I asked them.

"Here's the deal," I said. "If parents educate themselves about childbirth, they can make choices that lower their chances of having a traumatic birth. I also think every parent should meet with a childbirth educator at least once, to practice hands-on skills for comfort measures for childbirth. What kind of class could I offer that parents might find appealing?"

"Hmm," one of them said. "What if you offered a class that was part online, and part in person? Maybe they could meet as a group the first time, then continue meeting weekly online, like this?" (I was hosting the focus group using a video chat).

Everyone agreed. Then someone added, "Yeah! Then maybe the class could meet in real life one last time to practice their skills together!"

Inspired by their idea, I threw up a registration page with the type of class they'd envisioned. Within a few days, two couples signed up. I ended up spending the rest of 2018 working with local families, tweaking the curriculum, getting it just right. I decided to focus the class on learning about evidence based care, practicing comfort measure skills for labor, and teaching the partners and the birthing people how to advocate for themselves in the hospital.

One of my main goals for the parents who took my class was for them to feel empowered in their birth, no matter what type of birth they had. The first families who took the class told me they were experiencing just that! Whether they chose an unmedicated birth, a birth with an epidural, a home birth, a hospital birth, or a Cesarean—or even if their birth went entirely differently than they'd planned—they came back and told me they felt like their choices were informed and empowered.

Unfortunately, I was so distracted by teaching parents to advocate for themselves, that I temporarily forgot that sometimes there is nothing, absolutely nothing, I could do to help expecting parents avoid abuse from the health care system 100% of the time. A few weeks before my canoe trip with Dan, one of my former childbirth class students had texted me, sending me a photo of her new baby and thanking me for everything she'd learned in my class. But then she mentioned that an obstetrician performed a forced vaginal exam on her during labor. I could tell it had really traumatized her.

When I read her story, I got chills. Then I started crying.

I spent the rest of the day wandering around, restless, unable to sit still.

Would we never see change? What would it take for providers and nurses to learn that *no*, you don't just do a vaginal exam without the patient's explicit, freely given consent? When would they start seeing women as more than just a birth canal?

I knew, intuitively, that part of the solution was teaching medical students and nursing students about the importance of patient autonomy and evidence based care before they got out into the real world. And I'd done a bit of that—I continued teaching the "Babies Are Not Pizzas" college class for two years after I left my full-time job at the university. The pay was ridiculously low (welcome to the life of an adjunct!), and almost not worth it given the time commitment, but I continued teaching anyway. The two days per week that I sat in a classroom with the college students, discussing childbirth, were some of my favorite teaching moments, ever. The transformation from the beginning of the semester, when the students were so afraid of birth—to the end of the semester, when they were excited about the possibility of giving birth and firmly on the side of patient autonomy and evidence based care—was amazing.

On my final day of teaching last December, we gathered together to take a group photo. Afterward, as they lingered in the classroom, reluctant to leave, the students asked me if I was teaching next year, because they had friends who wanted to take my class.

"I would love to teach your friends next year!" I said. "But I've decided to take some time off from teaching to write a book."

I explained that a book about childbirth was something that I'd been thinking about doing for a long time, but I needed to carve out space and time in which to write. The students were disappointed that I wouldn't be around next year, but they were incredibly excited about the book, and asked if they could be among the first to read it when I finished.

Now, rowing down the creek with Dan, ten months had passed since my goodbye to my students, and even though I'd made time for writing by quitting the adjunct position, I was still struggling with the book. Originally, I was going to write an Evidence Based Birth® "Guide to Childbirth," starting with my first birth story, adding a bunch of evidence based information, and featuring case studies of why it's important to do things like hire a doula, educate yourself, pick the right provider, etc. I imagined my book up there on the library shelf, next to all the other pregnancy books—maybe with a cooler cover, definitely not the stereotypical blue and pink, but up there with those books, anyway.

After nine months of work, I sent the draft of my "Guide to Childbirth" book to some people I trusted to see what they thought. Most of them told me that they liked it.

But one of them, Aza, asked me to give her a call.

"The whole book felt disjointed," she said. "I just didn't connect with it as a reader."

I was disappointed, but I asked if there was anything she did connect with.

"The *yes* parts," Aza said, "had to do with your story. I kept turning the page, wondering what was going to happen next. I got emotionally involved. It was so powerful, especially when you combined it with the research evidence. Can't you just focus on telling your story, and weave the data around that?"

"Okay," I said. "But isn't that self-centered?"

"Look, Rebecca," she said. "Sometimes people have interesting lives. That doesn't mean you're self-centered. Tell your story."

"Okay," I said. "I'll think about it."

The day I talked with Aza, I sat down on my back porch and deleted most of my book draft.

And I sat there, and I looked out the window, and I thought. I thought about how there was no point in creating a how-to guide for parents until the health care system—until the culture of hospital staff—changed. Until health care workers respected the *right* of expecting families to choose evidence based options, my dream—that when my children gave birth themselves, evidence based care would be the norm—could not be realized.

I thought about how change happens.

And how does change happen?

The answer was right there, in a book I'd recently read by Dr. Stephen Pinker, a professor at Harvard University. In *Better Angels of Our Nature,* all about the decline of violence, Dr. Pinker examines the major human rights advances in the history of humankind.[160] He explains the forces behind massive changes like the end of slavery, the Civil Rights movement, the end of forced child labor, and women's suffrage—and how these changes happened.

As it turns out, culture change doesn't happen when we share data, or statistics, or evidence.

Instead, change happens when people realize that the people whose rights are being violated are human beings, just like them.

And often, that happens when we read stories.

Dr. Pinker theorizes that some of the biggest advances in human rights were partially due to the invention of the printing press and the expansion of literacy. That's because when we read a book, and we step inside the mindset of another person for a little while, we experience events the way someone else experienced them. We develop a heightened sense of empathy. We start to care.

What if, like Aza said, I should tell my story?

I knew my situation was unique in that it's highly unlikely that other insiders—nurses and doctors and midwives and professors in the system—will ever truly be able to speak up. Krysta Dancy, who had taught me so much about secondary trauma, had also informed me that there is a sort of "mythology of abusive institutions," where people on the inside believe that they can't speak up for several reasons. First, the cost is too high—it's too risky and dangerous. You could lose your job, be sued, and your whole family could be adversely affected. Second, the situation you were in was "not that bad." Others thought what was happening behind closed doors was acceptable, and if you tell the truth about what's happening there, you're being stupid and whiny. Third, people think it's futile. "It's not going to do any good to speak up, so why bother?"

I'd be lying if I said I didn't have any of these thoughts running through my mind.

This mythology of institutions—that what's happening in the organization is "not that bad," or that it's too risky or pointless to speak up—well, Krysta told me that sometimes this mythology is true, and sometimes it's not. But regardless, it's a story we tell ourselves to prevent us from speaking up about trauma and abuse.

In the end, our silence allows the trauma to continue. To affect generation after generation of nurses, midwives, doctors, doulas. And parents.

I'd never told my full, complete story to anyone. In fact, Dan and Cristen and a few immediate family members were the only people in the world who knew all of the crazy events I'd experienced over the course of the past decade. Always the introvert, I'd kept most of my life completely private, even when I became a public figure in the birth world. I was silent about the fact that I had two home births. I was silent about the fact that I hired a direct-entry midwife. I was silent about the fact that I was afraid to seek hospital care when I went past 42 weeks. I was silent about the racism happening in hospitals in my community. I was silent about the true reason for quitting my job. I was silent when I received countless emails and messages from women who'd been unnecessarily traumatized during their births.

But now, I am in the weirdest, most incredible, most bizarre situation of being entirely free. Dependent on no one person for my salary. Responsible to no one except to families around the world, who were still so desperately trying to get evidence based care inside broken health care systems. And what did they need me to do?

That night, after our trip down the river, Dan and I started our bedtime routine with Clara, Henry, and Susie. Once snack time was over, we raced them up the stairs, feigning that we were too slow to beat them (perhaps we were, though). At the top of the stairs, Henry blocked the stairway with his arms and yelled, "What's the password!!"

"Henry loves Mommy and Daddy!" we responded in unison, and the gate opened.

After brushing teeth, the kids got their pajamas on, and we read books with Henry and Susie, while Clara settled into her rocking chair to read her own book—she was reading through the Harry Potter series for the second time. (They grow up so fast.)

Then, one by one, we tucked the younger two into bed. After saying prayers and talking about what we were thankful for, we sang their favorite lullabies. Henry requested "Twinkle, Twinkle," and Susie asked for "Baby Mine."

I cuddled with Susie, per her usual request. As we laid there, and I stroked her hair, and we gazed into each other's eyes, she asked, "Mommy, will you tell me a story?"

"Yes," I said, and smiled. "Let me tell you a story about the night you were born."

Epilogue

THE WHOLE TIME I wrote this book, I imagined I was sitting in a coffee shop with you! Talking to you, telling you my story. So now, it's your turn to ask questions of me. You're looking at me from across the table, leaning forward, and you're probably asking, "Rebecca, but what can *I* do?"

Maybe you're fired up about the state of childbirth care in your hospital or community, and you want to create change, but you're not sure how. Or maybe you're anxious about your status as a patient in the health care system—and you're wondering, "How can I navigate this system and get the best care?"

On the next few pages, I've laid out some words of advice for you, depending on which situation you're in right now. Also, if you'd like even more information, for each section there is a corresponding video message waiting for you at Evidence Based Birth® website.

Maybe you've experienced a traumatic birth your-self. [evidencebasedbirth.com/trauma] If so, this book might have impacted you emotionally or even made you cry. Take some time today to care for yourself and process everything you've just read. Go on a walk or step outside. Take some deep breaths. Journal, meditate, exercise, or talk with a trusted friend or therapist.

Also, I want to tell you I'm sorry about what happened to you. It's not your fault. Please, focus on healing yourself. If you think you're having symptoms of post-traumatic stress (such as recurrent nightmares, flashbacks, intense emotional memories, avoidance of reminders of the trauma, emotional numbness, and being easily irritated), I'd highly recommend professional counseling with a therapist who specializes in PTSD, and who understands that PTSD can be associated with birth. There is a period of plasticity after a trauma when it is possible to get treatment that will help you re-arrange your thoughts about what happened to you, and help you cope with the memories and the aftermath of trauma. But even if it's been years, ther-apy can still help. One promising therapy for birth trauma is eye movement desensitization and reprocessing, or EMDR, which comes highly recommended by the therapists in the field. Remember, trauma doesn't go away on its own. It's got to be processed. The good news is, healing is absolutely possible.

Also, if you're planning on having more children in the future, please know that you can have an empowering birth following a traumatic one. I've met many, many families who were motivated by a negative experience to seek more sup-portive care the second time around. Find a compassionate, skilled provider. Hire a doula. Get educated. Get your birth plan and back-up plans ready. You can do this! You can feel supported and empowered in this next birth, no matter what type of birth it ends up being!

Maybe you're pregnant right now, or planning to have a baby in the future. [evidencebasedbirth.com/pregnant] And maybe you're thinking, "Oh no. I don't know if I've got the right provider or hospital." Well, if you're not pregnant yet, you've got tons of time to pick out the best place and provider for you. And if you're pregnant now, there's still time to educate yourself and build an amazing support team! Remember Cristen? She switched providers and hospitals on her second-to-last day of pregnancy! Other people I know have fired their provider *during labor*!

It's critical that you gather a team of people around you whom you can trust. When you think about your care situation, ask yourself, "What does my provider *routinely do?*" *not*, "Will they make an exception for my birth plan?" If they routinely induce *all* of their patients at 39 weeks, "require" vaginal exams (plus membrane sweeping) starting at 37 weeks, have a high Cesarean rate, have violated women's rights during childbirth in the past, or routinely start predicting a "big baby" in the beginning of your third trimester, then that's the kind of care that you're almost guaranteed to get. If you see any of these red flags, or you feel uncomfortable at all, my advice to you is run away from them, as fast as possible, and find someone else!

"But how do I know if they've committed obstetric violence in the past?" you might be asking. Well, that's easy enough to find out. Join a local birth or mother's group on social media, and ask the doulas and mothers in the group, "I need to hear your honest opinion. My OB/midwife practice name is so-and-so. Have you ever seen anyone from their practice coerce someone in their care during pregnancy or labor, or in any way disrespect a patient?" Chances are, some people will be willing to speak up and tell you if they've witnessed your provider at a birth, and what those experiences were like. Doulas, in particular, are magical! I highly recommend hiring a doula. They see everything, in every hospital in town, with nearly every provider and almost every nurse. They've seen amazing providers who practice safe and ethical care, horrible providers who cut episiotomies on every patient without asking permission, and everything in between. When you're interviewing doulas, ask if they will be honest with you about your provider! (Some may be reluctant to say anything critical about providers or hospitals—if they won't tell you their honest opinion, find other doulas who will). And remember, if your providers "rotate call" in their practice, this means that even if you've chosen a "good" provider, there's a chance you could get a "bad" one at your actual birth. Make sure you're with an OB or midwife practice that only has "good" ones!

Finally, please educate yourself! Unfortunately, I've met a lot of expecting parents who think they don't need to take a childbirth class. Maybe they think their doula can protect them, or maybe they think they can use the Internet and create a sort of self-education program. This path is problematic for several reasons. First of all, doulas cannot educate you during labor about all of your choices—when you're in labor, you're going to be in "labor land," focusing internally on your contractions. It's selling both of you short to think your doula can do their job well if you haven't done the work to inform yourself about the birth process and your options in various scenarios. Second, news flash: Much of the information on the Internet is wrong! As the founder of Evidence Based Birth®, I am often horrified by the outdated and inaccurate information I see, even on reputable, popular websites. Third, how many births have you attended? Your partner? Zero? One or two? You probably don't have the experience to know how to navigate the system and deal with the power hierarchy in labor and delivery, how to speak up for yourself, or what comfort measures to use during the different stages of labor. But it is entirely possible to learn how to do these things in a really good childbirth class. Go find one! One word of caution: some classes just teach you "what to expect in the hospital." That's not good enough. You need to find a class that teaches you practical advocacy techniques, comfort measure skills, and the evidence behind all your choices.

What if you're a partner, doula, nurse, midwife, or a physician who's witnessed trauma in the labor and delivery setting? [evidencebasedbirth.com/witness] I'm going to be frank with you. You probably need to see a therapist! Seriously! We need to destigmatize therapy! (I love it whenever one of my friends casually mentions, "Sure, I can do that when I get back from my therapy appointment," or "I was just telling my therapist the other day . . ." What a great way of modeling self-care!)

Here's the deal. I want you to have a long and fulfilling career. We need you! I've seen way too many professionals step away or leave birth work entirely because of secondary trauma. Don't let that happen to you. Take action and find a therapist today. And if you do have to step away, that's okay, too. I totally understand that you have to take care of yourself, even if it means taking a break from work in the childbirth field.

What if you realized, after reading Chapter Eight, "Woke," that you are part of perpetuating a system of racism? [evidencebasedbirth.com/woke] I started on my journey of working toward a more just world roughly five years ago. I'd love to invite you to join me in this process! Here are a few simple ways to get started:

First, realize that whether you mean to be or not, you are part of the problem—your privileges and advantages are a direct result of other people being unfairly disadvantaged and oppressed. Take the Implicit Bias tests at Harvard's implicit. harvard.edu website. Download the handout by Peggy McIntosh, called "White Privilege: Unpacking the Invisible Knapsack" (available for free at many websites),[161] and take note of the unearned privileges that you experience. I also highly recommend reading the book *Waking Up White: And Finding Myself in the Story of Race* by Debby Irving.[162]

Next, begin reading works by Black authors in the field of social justice. It's important that you do the work of educating yourself by using resources that have already been created, because it's oppressive to ask Black people to personally teach you about racism. There are so many books out there, but some that have been particularly impactful to me include *Why Are All the Black Kids Sitting Together in the Cafeteria* by Dr. Beverly Daniel Tatum,[163] *Incidents in the Life of a Slave Girl,* by Harriet Ann Jacobs,[164] and *Between the World and Me* by Ta-Nehisi Coates.[165]

Then, make sure you follow, support, and donate to Black organizations in the field of maternal health or social justice.

Black and Brown people are survivors—they are resilient, and they absolutely know what needs to be done to reduce disparities and improve the health of their people. They do not need us to save them! Instead, we need to let them lead the way, while we listen to their voices and support their work. Some notable birth-related social justice organizations include Mothering Justice, Black Mamas Matter, Mamatoto Village, Uzazi Village, Commonsense Childbirth, Black Women Birthing Justice, SisterSong, and the Changing Woman Initiative. And find out who is doing similar work local to you—there are so many people out there providing this hard, valuable service with little acknowledgment or support from the larger community.

Finally, don't stop. The journey of understanding white privilege and helping untangle the racism in our society is a lifelong process. I am five years along, and I am constantly learning new things about white supremacy culture and my role in racism. Also, don't expect to be perfect. (Surprisingly, in my readings, I found out that "perfectionism," which I suffer from, is considered a feature of white culture!) I've learned that in doing this work, I'm going to mess up. When I make a mistake, my goal is to acknowledge that I was wrong and work to make things better.

What if you're a professional who is stuck in a broken system, similar to how I felt trapped? [evidencebasedbirth. com/trapped] Maybe you're a "renegade midwife" or "rogue physician" or "troublemaking nurse," feeling demoralized and worn down from years of trying to protect your patients' autonomy or promote the midwifery model of care without losing your job. Maybe you're a doula, just trying to survive each birth, hoping that *this time* you won't see obstetric violence. What hope or words of advice can I give to you?

First of all, I want to say I am so sorry. I know it can feel horrible to stand by and watch while patients and their families—people you care about—are harmed by non-evidence-based and disrespectful care. Some days you want to quit, but you can't. Some days you go home and cry. It can be brutal.

The good news is, it's not all bad. Things *are* getting better in some aspects of childbirth care, albeit at a slower rate than many of us would like. Cesarean rates have been in the national spotlight in the last few years, and many hospitals are implementing quality improvement projects to lower the rate of preventable Cesareans. For people who do have Cesareans, their care is improving also. Ten years ago, doing skin-to-skin with your baby in the operating room was out of the question. Now, it's common in operating rooms around the world.

Also, as more celebrities hire midwives to attend their births (think Mila Kunis, Jennifer Connelly, and Hilary Duff), it's becoming more vogue to hire a midwife! Existing laws are being updated and new laws are being passed to provide more autonomy to nurse-midwives and certified professional midwives. In fact, the year I released this book, my state finally passed a bill that legalized certified professional midwives, so that home birth with direct-entry midwives will no longer take place underground!

Of course, there's still so much work to do. And the work revolves not only around evidence based care, but also respecting people's autonomy in birth. In fact, I see this as the primary battle that we face. Because until health care workers respect a pregnant parent's right to make decisions about their care—the right to informed consent and refusal—families won't be able to actually get the evidence based options they so desperately want.

In looking for solutions for you, the most helpful resource I found was a book I mentioned earlier called *Better Angels of Our Nature* by Dr. Steven Pinker.[166] Dr. Pinker teaches that, with any type of violence, there are three parties involved: 1) the victim, 2) the aggressor, and 3) the bystander.

Odds are a lot of you reading this right now are bystanders. So, let me tell you a secret. One way to reduce violence is for bystanders to help humanize the victims. Categorization, which *de*humanizes people under labels, is dangerous because it normalizes prejudice and makes it easier to carry out violent behaviors on the categorized group. As Dr. Pinker says, "Human sympathy can be turned on or off depending on how another person is categorized." What a powerful statement! We need to figure out how to get health care workers' minds reoriented so they consistently remember that the people in the birth room are individuals and fellow human beings. So expecting parents are not "The Ruptured Membranes in Room 520" or "The Labor in Room 521," but "Rebecca and Dan" or "Chaundrise and Ezekiel."

Another way that bystanders can help is by stigmatizing violence, bullying, and coercion in the labor and delivery unit so these actions become seen as repugnant. Right now, in many places, these actions are still normalized! Dr. Pinker writes about all of the horrific behaviors that some dominant humans enjoyed in the past (or at the very least, tolerated without speaking up), that are now viewed with disgust: animal abuse, hangings, lynchings, torture, hate crimes, child neglect, rape, and domestic violence. Once these things became stigmatized (believe it or not, they didn't used to be stigmatized!), they became social taboos and eventually criminalized.

Think about it. How can you make it taboo to treat pregnant women disrespectfully, coercively, or violently? Well, you need to speak up and use your voice! If you see obstetric violence, hold the line and say, "Stop! They did not consent!" Put an end to it at once! You can also use other tools to stigmatize obstetric violence, such as writing incident reports or formal letters of complaint, educating the other people on your unit about the definition of obstetric violence, scheduling a meeting with the unit supervisor, or going "up the chain of command."

Remember that violence can only continue *if bystanders let it continue.* Researchers call the silence of bystanders the "spiral of silence" or "pluralistic ignorance." Within this spiral, people who witness harmful behaviors either keep their mouths shut or sometimes even assist the aggressor, motivated by the thought that "Nobody else is saying anything, so it can't be wrong, right?" But, as Dr. Pinker says, "Pluralistic ignorance is a house of cards." All it takes is one person, or maybe two, and the false consensus that "It's okay to check her cervix without asking permission" or "It's okay to pressure her into giving birth on her back" will implode.

Listen, I know it's hard—incredibly hard—to be the lone voice, the only bystander willing to speak up. And I don't want you to necessarily do this by yourself, because it's very risky. Alone, you risk ostracism and potentially even losing your job (yes, this is an actual risk, and I've seen it happen to people before). It's critical that you mobilize your friends, your coworkers, or others to join you in stigmatizing and speaking up about forced and coerced procedures, disrespectful care, and non-evidence based care in childbirth. Can you imagine, if every single labor and delivery nurse in the country stood up and said, "We will no longer tolerate our patients being bullied or coerced or lied to or treated in any other disrespectful way." My guess is, if that happened, disrespectful care would vanish overnight!

But, how can you do that? How can you get allies? I would highly recommend you reach out to all the new people on your unit—the new nurses, the students, the new residents. Often, they are the most receptive to new ideas. Offer to teach them about evidence based care, physiologic birth, non-pharmacologic comfort measures, and informed consent and refusal.

Also, I've just provided you with another tool you can use with anyone. This book. Share it! If you're feeling brave, create a book club, or talk about what you read in this book openly at the nurse's station! If you're worried about being seen as a renegade, then anonymously leave a copy in the call room or staff bathroom, with relevant passages highlighted! (In my former life as a staff nurse, we called this "toilet training!")

What if you're a professional, and you're realizing that you might have violated patients' autonomy in the past, through conscious or subconscious acts of coercion, pressure, bullying, lying, or forced care? [evidencebasedbirth.com/better] I know you're out there, because I've met many professionals who hang their head in shame and tell me, "I was that nurse," or, "I was that doctor," or, "I was that midwife." Look. You can't change the past. You didn't know better then. You were trapped in a cycle of trauma. You witnessed trauma, you were trained how to do it, and you perpetuated it.

But you know better now, so now it's your responsibility to do better. Educate yourself on how to provide true informed consent and trauma-informed care. Humanize your clients. Talk with your peers about what you're learning. Network with and get to know the doulas and home birth midwives in your community, so that you can begin to form family-centered care teams in which everyone is valued. And most importantly, work with your students and trainees to ensure that they don't repeat the mistakes you made in the past.

Finally, what if you're a student in the medical, midwifery, or nursing field? [evidencebasedbirth.com/student] Good news . . . you are our future! You also happen to be my hope, and my inspiration. You will be there by my family's side when Clara, Henry, and Susie are creating families of their own. I can't wait to meet you someday!

My dream for you, dear student, is that you find a way to be an advocate for evidence based, compassionate care for all the humans you come across in your clinical practice. This won't be an easy path, as it's definitely the path less traveled at this point in history. It will take time for you to learn how to promote patient autonomy in a medical culture that doesn't always hold the same values as you. In the meantime, you can learn some really good, respectful communication skills. I know these skills are not always taught sufficiently in school. So, to get started, I recommend reading the book *Mastering Respectful Confrontation* by Joe Weston.[167]

One word of advice. If you haven't chosen a program yet, be picky where you choose to go to medical school, nursing school, or residency. Your first choice should be to find an environment already practicing evidence based care, one that integrates midwives, nurses, doulas, and physicians into a team in which all professions are valued and families are at the center of care. Also, importantly, when you pick your first job, find a workplace in which your immediate supervisor is a caring person who models compassionate, respectful patient care. If you can't find these places, or you find yourself in a situation that's the opposite, do your best to lead by example. Show others what high-quality childbirth care can really be like. Find friends and coworkers who will join forces with you. You have the power to help us close a chapter on preventable trauma being perpetuated from generation to generation.

And finally, I wanted to give one last piece of advice. **For those of you who are afraid**—anxious about birth, or hard conversations, or retaliation, or change, or the future—let me give you some final direction. I charge you to follow in my footsteps. You don't need to get your PhD, or start a blog, or quit your job, in order to create change—that's not what I'm talking about. But I do want you to find your courage. Face your fears head on, and do the right thing. Speak the truth in love. And know that you are not alone! We're all in this together!

Take heart, and envision this: long after you and I are gone, future generations will look back and remember what happened here. They will remember that we were the ones who stood up and said:

No more. We will no longer tolerate poor care and preventable harm in childbirth. A new cycle of empowerment and compassion during childbirth begins with us, and it begins today.

Thank You for Reading This Book!

I WOULD LOVE TO HEAR from you! If you'd like to drop me a message, simply email info@evidencebasedbirth. com, and put "Book message" in the subject line.

Also, if you're willing, I would like to ask a small favor of you. Would you post an honest review of *Babies Are Not Pizzas*? All you have to do is go to the website where you bought the book (or the website for the store) and submit the review. Reviews are a great way for parents and professionals to discover this book and decide if it will be of benefit to them.

Thank you so much! I look forward to hearing from you and/or reading your review!

—Rebecca

Resources

EVIDENCE BASED BIRTH®
FREE RESOURCES

EVIDENCE BASED BIRTH® (**www.evidencebasedbirth. com**) exists to raise the quality of childbirth care globally by making research evidence on childbirth publicly accessible to families and professionals. Evidence Based Birth® offers a variety of free resources to assist you:

Evidence Based Birth® Signature Articles, available on our blog, are peer-reviewed articles covering the evidence on a variety of childbirth topics. Free one-page summary handouts are also available. To get started, you may want to read one of our top 5 most popular articles:

- Evidence on: Vitamin K (ebbirth.com/vitamink)
- Evidence on: Due Dates (ebbirth.com/duedates)
- Evidence on: Group B Strep (ebbirth.com/groupbstrep)

- Evidence on: Big Babies (ebbirth.com/bigbaby)
- Evidence on: Eye Ointment (ebbirth.com/eyeointment)

The **Evidence Based Birth® Podcast** is available on a variety of platforms, including iTunes, Stitcher, and Spotify. New episodes drop each Wednesday!

The **Evidence Based Birth® Email Newsletter** offers a variety of free benefits, including a crash course on evidence based care, weekly updates, and announcements about webinars and other events. You can join by filling out the form at **www.evidencebasedbirth.com.**

Follow **Evidence Based Birth® on Social Media** via Facebook (@evidencebasedbirth), Instagram (@ebbirth), Twitter (@birthevidence), and YouTube (@evidencebasedbirth).

Don't forget to check out our free **YouTube series on Pain Management during Labor and Natural Induction Methods!**

EVIDENCE BASED BIRTH®
PREMIUM RESOURCES

If you'd like to take your learning to the next level, we offer the following premium resources:

Parents:

For parents, we offer the Evidence Based Birth® Childbirth Class in communities around the world. To find a class near you, search our directory at **www.evidencebasedbirth.com/events.**

Our Evidence Based Birth® Instructors also offer Savvy Birth workshops and special prenatal visits for their clients. To find an

Instructor near you, visit **www.directory.evidencebasedbirth. com.**

Professionals:

Consider joining the EBB Professional Membership for professionals who are committed to changing childbirth care. Visit **www.evidencebasedbirth.com/membership.**

If you would like to teach our content, we accept applications into the EBB Instructor program twice yearly. Learn more at **www.evidencebasedbirth.com/instructor.**

Attend a live continuing education workshop on topics such as Comfort Measures, Savvy Birth Pro, Due Dates, or Home Birth Transfers. Search our events at **www.evidence-basedbirth.com/events.**

Incorporate Evidence Based Birth® curriculum into your university, college, training program, or nursing unit via our EBB Higher Ed program. Learn more at **https://evidence-basedbirth.com/join-highered/.**

Acknowledgments

THERE ARE SO MANY people who have supported me and Evidence Based Birth® over the years. First, I'd like to thank Dan Dekker, who, from the very first moments of EBB, has been 100% supportive and on board. I am so grateful that you are my partner! Thank you to our beautiful children, Clara, Henry, and Susie, for so patiently allowing EBB to be part of our family's life. For the past seven years, you've done a great job of listening to your mom talk non-stop about birth, never once rolling your eyes or being embarrassed! Right? Thank you also to my beloved sister, Shannon, for everything . . . you know what I'm talking about! Cristen Pascucci!! I have to thank you for your friendship, your brilliant medical editing (including the substantial edits you made to this book), and your passion for supporting survivors of obstetric violence.

I'd also like to thank the entire EBB team: Katie Pontone, Cat LaPlante, Anna Bertone, Joseph Pareja, Divine Cleto, Chante Perryman, and Victoria Wilson. Thank you also to Sarah Wylie, who gave me permission to share her birth story in this book; your generous spirit and your heart for postpartum families has had a huge impact on my life. Thank you to our customers, especially our Professional Members and Instructors, who have supported the work we do and provided me with constant encouragement and inspiration. Thank you to my research mentors, Debra, Terry, Misook, and the rest of the RICH Heart Team, for molding me into a research scientist. You believed in me and never stopped caring about me, even when I left academia to pursue advocacy work and entrepreneurship! Thank you to my midwife, Karen Brown, whose evidence based, family-centered care inspired me to share what I'd learned about midwifery with the world. Thank you for all the service you so selflessly provided to families in our state who wanted to birth outside the system. I'd also like to express my thanks to Sarah and Kenny VanderBent, Dawn Thompson, Briana, Caroline Malatesta, Shane and Jocelyn Sams, Jodi Hume, Krysta Dancy, Ngozi Tibbs, Cheryl Beck, and Aza Nedhari.

I couldn't have done all of the work that I documented in this book without a loving, supportive family. Thank you to my family, especially my dad, Vincent DeYoung, author and attorney and our kids' "Pop Pop," who has critiqued my writing since I was in middle school! Special thanks go to my mom, Carol DeYoung, nurse and medical missionary and grandma extraordinaire, who has been my sounding board for so many of my ruminations about all things birth. And thank you to my other DeYoung siblings and siblings-in-law—Donna, Cindy, John, Krista, Ryan, and Mary, and to my Dekker parents-in-law, Dave and Peggy, and siblings-in-law, Mike, Lisa,

Nick, Beth, and Greg, for always loving and supporting Dan and me.

Finally, thank you to all the college and graduate students who have influenced my work over the years. Whether you sat in one of my large lecture halls in pathopharmacology, or worked with me one-on-one in research internships, or sat in "Babies Are Not Pizzas" and hashed out these topics with me, thank you for being my inspiration and hope for the future.

Endnotes

Chapter One

1. Smyth, R. M., Markham, C., and Dowswell, T. (2013). Amniotomy for shortening spontaneous labour. Cochrane Database Syst Rev, Issue 6. Art. No.: CD006167.

2. ACOG Committee Opinion No. 766 (2019). Approaches to limit intervention during labor and birth. Obstet Gynecol, 133: e164–73.

3. U.S. Food and Drug Administration: Pitocin® drug label. Accessed online May 27, 2019. Available at: https://www.accessdata.fda.gov/drugsatfda_docs/label/2014/018261s031lbl.pdf

4. Hannah, M. E., Ohlsson, A., Farine, D., et al. (1996). Induction of labor compared with expectant management for prelabor rupture of the membranes at term. TERMPROM Study Group. N Engl J Med, 334: 1005–10.

5. Anim-Somuah, M., Smyth, R. M., Cyna, A. M., et al. (2018). Epidural versus non-epidural or no analgesia for pain management in labour. Cochrane Database Syst Rev, Issue 5. Art. No.: CD000331.

6. Lawrence, A., Lewis, L., Hofmeyr, G. J., et al. (2013). Maternal positions and mobility during first stage labour. Cochrane Database Syst Rev, Issue 10. Art. No.: CD003934.

7. Neczypor, J. L. and Holley, S. L. (2017). Providing evidence-based care during the golden hour. Nurs Womens Health, 21(6): 462–472.

8. Beck, C. T., Driscoll, J., and Watson, S. (2013). *Traumatic Childbirth*. Abingdon, Oxon: Routledge.

9. Hodnett, E. D. (2002). Pain and women's satisfaction with the experience of childbirth: A systematic review. Am J Obstet Gynecol, 186(5): S160–72.

Chapter Two

10. ACOG Committee Opinion No. 763 (2018). Optimizing postpartum care. Obstet Gynecol, 131: e140–50.

11. Sackett, D. L., Rosenberg, W. M., Gray, J. A., et al. (1996). Evidence based medicine: what it is and what it isn't. BMJ (Clinical research ed.), 312(7023): 71–72.

12. Institute of Medicine (2001). Committee on Quality of Health Care in America. Crossing the quality chasm: A new health system for the 21st century: National Academies Press. Access the e-book for free: http://books.nap.edu/openbook.php?record_id=10027

13. Ciardulli, A., Saccone, G., Anastasio, H., et al. (2017). Less-restrictive food intake during labor in low- risk singleton pregnancies: A systematic review and meta-analysis. Obstet Gynecol, 129(3): 473–480.

14. Lawrence, A., Lewis, L., Hofmeyr, G. J., et al. (2013). Maternal positions and mobility during first stage labour. Cochrane Database Syst Rev, Issue 10. Art. No.: CD003934.

15. Portz, S., Schmidt, M. and Weitz, M. (2016). Lying down after premature rupture of the membranes in term singleton pregnancies: An evidence-based recommendation? Z Geburtshilfe Neonatol, 220(5): 200–206.

16. Dawood, F., Dowswell, T., and Quenby, S. (2013). Intravenous fluids for reducing the duration of labour in low risk nulliparous women. Cochrane Database Syst Rev, Issue 6. Art. No.: CD007715.

17. Kujawa-Myles, S., Noel-Weiss, J., Dunn, S., et al. (2015). Maternal intravenous fluids and postpartum breast changes: A pilot observational study. Int Breastfeed J, 10: 18.

18. Noel-Weiss, J., Woodend, A. K., Peterson, W. E., et al. (2011). An observational study of associations among maternal fluids during parturition, neonatal output, and breastfed newborn weight loss. Int Breastfeed J, 6: 9.

19. Chantry, C. J., Nommsen-Rivers, L. A., Peerson, J. M., et al. (2011). Excess weight loss in first-born breastfed newborns relates to maternal intrapartum fluid balance. Pediatrics, 127(1): e171–9.

20. Watson, J., Hodnett, E., Armson, B. A., et al. (2012). A randomized controlled trial of the effect of intrapartum intravenous fluid management on breastfed newborn weight loss. J Obstet Gynecol Neonatal Nurs, 41(1): 24–32.

21. Alfirevic, Z., Devane, D., Gyte, G. M., et al. (2017). Continuous cardiotocography (CTG) as a form of electronic fetal monitoring (EFM) for fetal assessment during labour. Cochrane Database Syst Rev, Issue 2. Art. No.: CD006066.

22. Bugg, G. J., Siddiqui, F., and Thornton, J. G. (2013). Oxytocin versus no treatment or delayed treatment for slow progress in the first stage of spontaneous labour. Cochrane Database Syst Rev, Issue 6. Art. No.: CD007123.

23. Cluett, E. R., Pickering, R. M., Getliffe, K., et al. (2004). Randomised controlled trial of labouring in water compared with standard of augmentation for management of dystocia in first stage of labour. BMJ, 328: 314.

24. Simpson, K. R. and Knox, G. E. (2009). Oxytocin as a high-alert medication: Implications for perinatal patient safety. MCN Am J Matern Child Nurs, 34(1): 8–15.

25. Hannah, M. E., Ohlsson, A., Farine, D., et al. (1996). Induction of labor compared with expectant management for prelabor rupture of the membranes at term. TERMPROM Study Group. N Engl J Med, 334: 1005–10.

26. Imseis, H. M., Trout, W. C., and Gabbe, S. G. (1999). The microbiologic effect of digital cervical examination. Am J Obstet Gynecol, 180(3 Pt 1): 578–80.

27. Seaward, P. G., Hannah, M. E., Myhr, T. L., et al. (1997). International Multicentre Term Prelabor Rupture of Membranes Study: Evaluation of predictors of clinical chorioamnionitis and postpartum fever in patients with prelabor rupture of membranes at term. Am J Obstet Gynecol, 177(5): 1024–9.

28. Downe, S., Gyte, G. M. L., Dahlen, H. G., et al. (2013). Routine vaginal examinations for assessing progress of labour to improve outcomes for women and babies at term. Cochrane Database Syst Rev, Issue 7. Art. No.: CD010088.

29. Anim-Somuah, M., Smyth, R. M. D., Cyna, A. M., et al. (2018). Epidural versus non-epidural or no analgesia for pain management in labour. Cochrane Database Syst Rev, Issue 5. Art. No.: CD000331.

30. Shnider, S. M., Abboud, T. K., Artal, R., et al. (1983). Maternal catecholamines decrease during labor after lumbar epidural anesthesia. Am J Obstet Gynecol, 147(1): 13–5.

31. Shaw-Battista, J. (2017). Systematic review of hydrotherapy research: Does a warm bath in labor promote normal physiologic childbirth? J Perinat Neonatal Nurs, 31(4): 303–316.

32. Makvandi, S., Roudsari, R. L., Sadeghi, R., et al. (2015). Effect of birth ball on labor pain relief: A systematic review and meta-analysis. J Obstet Gynaecol Res, 41(11): 1679–86.

33. Declercq, E., Sakala, C., Corry, M. P., et al. (2002). Listening to mothers: Report of the first national U.S. survey of women's childbearing experiences. New York: Maternity Center Association.

34. Smith, C. A., Collins, C. T., Crowther, C. A., et al. (2011). Acupuncture or acupressure for pain management in labour. Cochrane Database Syst Rev, Issue 7. Art No.:CD009232.

35. Kaviani, M., Maghbool, S., Azima, S., et al. (2014). Comparison of the effect of aromatherapy with Jasminum officinale and Salvia officinale on pain severity and labor outcome in nulliparous women. Iran J Nurs Midwifery Res, 19(6): 666–72.

36. Burns, E.E., Blamey, C., Ersser, S.J., et al. (2000). An investigation into the use of aromatherapy in intrapartum midwifery practice. J Altern Complement Med, 6(2): 141–7.

37. Smith, C. A., Levett, K. M., Collins C. T., et al. (2018). Massage, reflexology and other manual methods for pain management in labour. Cochrane Database Syst Rev, Issue 3. Art. No.: CD009290.

38. Smith, C. A., Levett, K. M., Collins, C. T. (2018). Relaxation techniques for pain management in labour. Cochrane Database Syst Rev, Issue 3. Art. No.: CD009514.

39. Gokyildiz Surucu, S. G., Ozturk, M., Vurgec, B. A., et al. (2018). The effect of music on pain and anxiety of women in labor during their first pregnancy: A study from Turkey. Complement Ther Clin Pract, 30: 96–102.

40. Pirdel, M. and Pirdel, L. (2009). Perceived environmental stressors and pain perception during labor among primiparous and multiparous women. J Reprod Infertil, 10(3): 217–223.

41. Lowe, N. K. (1996). The pain and discomfort of labor and birth. J Obstet Gynecol Neonatal Nurs, 25(1): 82–92.

42. Buckley, S. J. (2015). Executive summary of Hormonal Physiology of Childbearing: Evidence and implications for women, babies, and maternity care. J Perinat Educ, 24(3): 145–153.

43. Anderson, B. and Stone, S. (2013). *Best Practices in Midwifery*. New York: Springer.

44. McGrath, S. K. and Kennell, J. H. (2008). A randomized controlled trial of continuous labor support for middle-class couples: Effect on Cesarean delivery rates. Birth, 35(2): 92–7.

45. Nutter, E., Meyer, S., Shaw-Battista, J., et al. (2014). Water birth: An integrative analysis of peer-reviewed literature. J Midwifery Womens Health, 59(3): 286–319.

46. Vanderlaan, J., Hall, P. J., and Lewitt, M. (2018). Neonatal outcomes with water birth: A systematic review and meta-analysis. Midwifery, 59: 27–38.

47. Bovbjerg, M. L., Cheyney, M. and Everson, C. (2016). Maternal and newborn outcomes following water birth: The

Midwives Alliance of North America statistics project, 2004 to 2009 cohort. J Midwifery Womens Health, 61(1): 11–20.

48. Hagadorn, J., Guthri, E., Atkins, K.A., et al. (1997). Neonatal aspiration pneumonitis and endotracheal colonization with burkholderia picketti following home water birth. Pediatrics, 100(3S): 506.

49. Nguyen, S., Kuschel, C., Teele, R., et al. (2002). Water birth—a near-drowning experience. Pediatrics, 110(2 Pt 1): 411–3.

50. Gilbert, R. E. and Tookey, P. A. (1999). Perinatal mortality and morbidity among babies delivered in water: surveillance study and postal survey. BMJ, 319: 483.

51. Nagai, T., Sobajima, H., Iwasa, M., et al. (2003). Neonatal sudden death due to Legionella pneumonia associated with water birth in a domestic spa bath. J Clin Microbiol, 41(5): 2227–2229.

52. Collins, S. L., Afshar, B., Walker, J. T., et al. (2016). Heated birthing pools as a source of Legionnaires' disease. Epidemiol Infect, 144(4): 796–802.

53. ACOG Committee Opinion No. 679. (2016). Immersion in water during labor and delivery. Obstet Gynecol, 128: e231–6.

54. Gupta, J. K., Sood, A., Hofmeyr, G. J., et al. (2017). Position in the second stage of labour for women without epidural anaesthesia. Cochrane Database Syst Rev, Issue 5. Art. No.: CD002006.

55. Walker, C., Rodríguez, T., Herranz, A., et al. (2012). Alternative model of birth to reduce the risk of assisted vaginal delivery and perineal trauma. Int Urogynecol J, 23(9): 1249–56.

56. Lemos, A., Amorim, M. M., Dornelas de Andrade, A., et al. (2017). Pushing/ bearing down methods for the second stage of labour. Cochrane Database Syst Rev, Issue 3. Art. No.: CD009124.

57. Altman, M., Sandstrom, A., Petersson, G., et al. (2015). Prolonged second stage of labor is associated with low Apgar score. Eur J Epidemiol, 30(11): 1209–15.

58. Sandström, A., Altman, M., Cnattingius, S. (2017). Durations of second stage of labor and pushing, and adverse

neonatal outcomes: A population-based cohort study. J Perinatol, 37(3): 236–242.

59. ACOG, SMFM, Caughey, A. B., et al. (2014). Safe prevention of the primary cesarean delivery. Am J Obstet Gynecol, 210(3): 179–93.

60. Shaffer, B. L., Cheng, Y. W., Vargas, J. E., et al. (2011). Manual rotation to reduce cesarean delivery in persistent occiput posterior or transverse position. J Matern Fetal Neonatal Med, 24(1): 65–72.

61. Aflaifel, N. and Weeks, A. (2012). Push, pull, squeeze, clamp: 100 years of changes in the management of the third stage of labour as described by Ten Teachers. BMJ, 345: e8270.

62. Katheria, A. C., Lakshminrusimha, S., Rabe, H., et al. (2017). Placental transfusion: A review. J Perinatol, 37(2): 105–111.

63. Ashish, K. C., Rana, N., Malqvist, M., et al. (2017). Effects of delayed umbilical cord clamping vs. early clamping on anemia in infants at 8 and 12 months: A randomized clinical trial. JAMA Pediatr, 171(3): 264–270.

64. Mercer, J. S., Erickson-Owens, D. A., Deoni, S., et al. (2018). Effects of delayed cord clamping on 4-month ferritin levels, brain myelin content, and neurodevelopment: A randomized controlled trial. J Pediatr, 203: 266–272.e2.

65. McDonald, S. J., Middleton, P., Dowswell, T., et al. (2013). Effect of timing of umbilical cord clamping of term infants on maternal and neonatal outcomes. Cochrane Database Syst Rev, Issue 7. Art. No.: CD004074.

66. McDonald, S. J. (1996). Management in the third stage of labour [dissertation]. Perth: University of Western Australia.

67. Hutton and Hassan (2007). Late vs. early clamping of the umbilical cord in full-term neonates: Systematic review and meta-analysis of controlled trials. JAMA, 297(11): 1241–52.

68. Mercer, J. S., Erickson-Owens, D. A., Collins, J., et al. (2017). Effects of delayed cord clamping on residual placental blood volume, hemoglobin and bilirubin levels in term infants: A randomized controlled trial. J Perinatol, 37(3): 260–264.

69. Anderson, G. C., Radjenovic D., Chiu, S. H., et al. (2004). Development of an observational instrument to measure mother-infant separation post birth. J Nurs Meas, 12(3): 215–34.

70. Neczypor, J. L. and Holley, S. L. (2017). Providing evidence-based care during the golden hour. Nurs Womens Health, 21(6): 462–472.

71. Moore, E. R., Bergman, N., Anderson, G. C., et al. (2016). Early skin-to-skin contact for mothers and their healthy newborn infants. Cochrane Database Syst Rev, Issue 11. Art. No.: CD003519.

72. Bystrova, K., Ivanova, V., Edhborg, M., et al. (2009). Early contact versus separation: Effects on mother-infant interaction one year later. Birth, 36(2): 97–109.

Chapter Three

73. Buckley, S. J. (2015). Executive summary of Hormonal Physiology of Childbearing: Evidence and implications for women, babies, and maternity care. J Perinat Educ, 24(3): 145–153.

74. Davis-Floyd, R. (2018). *Ways of Knowing About Birth: Mothers, Midwives, Medicine, & Birth Activism: Selected Writings by Robbie Davis-Floyd and Colleagues*. Waveland Press, Inc. Long Grove, Illinois.

75. Varney, H. and Thompson, J. B. (2016). *The Midwife Said Fear Not: A History of Midwifery in the United States*. Springer Publishing Company, LLC, New York.

76. Martin, J. A., Hamilton, B. E., Osterman, M. J. K., et al. (2018). Births: Final Data for 2017. National Vital Statistics Reports, 67(8), Hyattsville, MD: National Center for Health Statistics.

77. Wren Serbin, J. and Donnelly, E. (2016). The impact of racism and midwifery's lack of racial diversity: A literature review. J Midwifery Womens Health, 61(6): 694–706.

78. Leavitt, J. W. (1986). *Brought to Bed: Childbearing in America, 1750 to 1950*. New York: Oxford University Press.

79. Scott, S. L. (1983). Grannies, mothers and midwives: An

examination of traditional Southern lay midwifery. Central Issues in Anthropology, 4 (2): 17–29.

80 McDermott, K. W., Elixhauser, A. and Sun, R. (2017). Trends in Hospital Inpatient Stays in the United States, 2005–2014. HCUP Statistical Brief #225; Agency for Healthcare Research and Quality, Rockville, MD. Available at: https://www.hcup-us.ahrq.gov/reports/statbriefs/sb225-Inpatient-US-Stays-Trends.pdf

81. Loftman, P. O. (2018). Revisiting an ugly past. Quickening, 49 (4): 10–11. Available at: http://www.midwife.org/acnm/files/ccLibraryFiles/Filename/000000007171/Final_Fall18Quickening.pdf

82. Leavitt, J. W. (1980). Birthing and anesthesia: The debate over Twilight Sleep. J Women Culture Society, 6(1): 147–164.

83. Leavitt, J. W. (2009). *Make Room for Daddy: The Journey from Waiting Room to Birthing Room.* University of North Carolina Press.

84. Stevenson, C. S., et al. (1958). Maternal deaths from obstetric anesthesia and analgesia: Can they be eliminated? Obstet Gynecol 8(1): 88–98.

85. Brazelton, T. B. (1961). Effects of maternal medication on the neonate and his behavior. J Pediatrics 58: 513–518.

86. D'Angelo, R., Smiley, R. M., Riley, E. T., et al. (2014). Serious complications related to obstetric anesthesia: The serious complication repository project of the Society for Obstetric Anesthesia and Perinatology. Anesthesiology, 120(6), 1505–1512.

87. Friedman, E. A. (1955). "Primigravid labor; a graphicostatistical analysis." Obstet Gynecol 6(6): 567– 589.

88. Zhang, J., Landy, H. J., Branch, D. W. et al and the Consortium on Safe Labor (2010). "Contemporary patterns of spontaneous labor with normal neonatal outcomes." Obstet Gynecol 116(6): 1281–1287.

89. Boyle, A., U. M. Reddy, H. J. Landy, et al. (2013). Primary cesarean delivery in the United States. Obstet Gynecol 122(1): 33–40.

90. Cunningham, F. G., Williams, J. W. (2010). *Williams Obstetrics*, 23rd ed. New York : McGraw-Hill.

91. Marzalik, P. R., Feltham, K. J., Jefferson, K., et al. (2018). Midwifery education in the U.S. - Certified Nurse-Midwife, Certified Midwife and Certified Professional Midwife. Midwifery, 60: 9–12.

92. ACOG Committee Opinion No. 476. (2011). Planned home birth. Obstet Gynecol, 117 (2 Pt 1): 425–8.

93. Newton, N. (1987). The fetus ejection reflex revisited. Birth, 14(2): 106–108.

Chapter Four

94. Leary, M. Why You Are Who You Are: Investigations into Human Personality. Available at: https://www.thegreatcourses.com/courses/why-you-are-who-you-are-investigations-into-human-personality.html

95. Kotter, J. P. and Cohen, D. S. (2002). *The Heart of Change: Real-Life Stories of How People Change Their Organizations.* Harvard Business School Press, MA.

96. Davis-Floyd, R. (2018). *Ways of Knowing About Birth: Mothers, Midwives, Medicine, & Birth Activism: Selected Writings by Robbie Davis-Floyd and Colleagues.* Waveland Press, Inc. Long Grove, Illinois.

97. Covey, S. R. (1989; 2004). *The 7 Habits of Highly Effective People: Powerful Lessons in Personal Change.* Free Press, New York, NY.

Chapter Five

98. Carter, M. (2019). Average U.S. Student Loan Debt Statistics. Credible. Available at: https://www.credible.com/blog/statistics/average-student-loan-debt-statistics/#average-debt-school-type

99. Association of American Medical Colleges (2018). Medical

Student Education: Debt, Costs, and Loan Repayment Fact Card. Available at: https://store.aamc.org/downloadable/download/ sample/sample_id/240/

100. Levy, S. (2017). Residents Salary and Debt Report. Medscape. Available at: https://www.medscape.com/slideshow/ residents-salary-and-debt-report-2017-6008931#3

101. American Academy of Family Physicians (2019). Hospital Credentialing and Privileging FAQs. Available at: https://www.aafp. org/practice-management/administration/privileging/credentialing-privileging-faqs.html

102. HealthLeaders Media Staff (2008). 'Disruptive Physician' Needs A Better Definition. Available at: https://www.healthleadersmedia. com/strategy/disruptive-physician-needs-better-definition

103. Reynolds, N.T. (2012). Disruptive physician behavior: Use and misuse of the label. Journal of Medical Licensure and Discipline, 98: 8–19.

104 .Wikipedia (2019). National Practitioner Data Bank. Available at: https://en.m.wikipedia.org/wiki/National_Practitioner_Data_Bank

105. Maguire, K. and Kirschenbaum, J., Suspension or Revocation of Hospital Privileges – Knowing Your Rights and What to Expect. Kirschenbaum & Kirschenbaum, P.C. Attorneys at Law. Available at: https://www.kirschenbaumesq.com/article/ pdf/002494-suspension-or-revocation-of-hospital-privileges.pdf

106. Indest, G. F. (2019). You Might Be A Disruptive Physician If . . .Avoiding the Disruptive Physician Label, The Health Law Firm. Available at: https://www.thehealthlawfirm.com/resources/ health-law-articles-and-documents/You-might-be-a-disruptive-physician-if-avoiding-the-disruptive-physician-label.html

107. Brill Legal Group, P. C. (2019). Disruptive Physician Defense Attorney, New York Disruptive Physician Defense Attorney. Available at: https://www.brill-legal.com/our-services/ health-care-law-attorneys/disruptive-physician-defense-attorney/

108. Weiss Zarett Brofman Sonnenklar & Levy, P.C. (2010). How the Title of "Disruptive Physician" Can Ruin Your Career and How to Avoid It, Bringing Experience & Dedication to Healthcare Law & Business Law, Firm News & Legal Alerts. Available at:

https://weisszarett.com/lawyer/2010/08/01/Healthcare-Law/How-the-Title-of-%E2%80%9CDisruptive-Physician%E2%80%9D-Can-Ruin-Your-Career-and-How-to-Avoid-It_bl31980.htm

109. Williams, T. K. (2012). "Understanding Internalized Oppression: A Theoretical Conceptualization of Internalized Subordination." Open Access Dissertations. 627. Available at: https://scholarworks.umass.edu/open_access_dissertations/627

110. Love, B. (2000). Developing a liberatory consciousness. In Adams, M., Blumenfield, W. J., Castañeda, R., et al. (Eds.), *Readings for Diversity and Social Justice* (2nd ed., pp. 470–474). New York, NY: Routledge.

111. Harari, Y. N. (2014) *Sapiens: A Brief History of Humankind.* Published in the U.K. by Harvill Secker First; published in Hebew in Israel in 2011 by Kinneret, Zmora-Bitan, Dvir.

112. Douglas, K. (2014). Nurses eat their own; Bullying and horizontal violence takes its toll. Aust Nurs Midwifery J, 21(8): 20–4.

113. Bambi, S., Foà, C., De Felippis, C., et al. (2018). Workplace incivility, lateral violence and bullying among nurses. A review about their prevalence and related factors. Acta Biomed, 89(6-S): 51–79.

114. Institute of Medicine (2001). Committee on Quality of Health Care in America. Crossing the quality chasm: A new health system for the 21st century: National Academies Press. Access the e-book for free: http://books.nap.edu/openbook.php?record_id=10027

115. Berwick, D. M. (2009). What 'patient-centered' should mean: Confessions of an extremist. Health Affairs, 28(S1): w555-w565.

Chapter Six

116. ACOG Committee Opinion No. 390 (2007; reaffirmed 2016). Ethical decision making in obstetrics and gynecology. Obstet Gynecol, 110: 1479–87.

117. De Bord, J. (2014). Informed Consent. Ethics in Medicine:

University of Washington School of Medicine. Available at: https:// depts.washington.edu/bioethx/topics/consent.html

118. Kukura, E. (2018). Obstetric Violence. The Georgetown Law Journal 106. Available at: https://georgetownlawjournal.org/ articles/261/obstetric-violence

119. LaBarre, Suzanne. (2013). Why we're turning off our comments. Popular Science. Available at: https://www.popsci.com/ science/article/2013-09/why-were-shutting-our-comments/

120. Anderson, A.A., Brossard, D., Scheufele, D. A., et al. (2013). The "nasty effect:" Online incivility and risk perceptions of emerging technologies. J Comput Mediat Commun, 19(3).

Chapter Seven

121. NobelPrize.org. (2019). George Bernard Shaw – Biographical. From Nobel Lectures, Literature 1901–1967, Editor Horst Frenz, Elsevier Publishing Company, Amsterdam, 1969. Available at: https://www.nobelprize.org/prizes/literature/1925/ shaw/biographical/

122. Khambalia, A. Z., Roberts, C. L., Nguyen, M., et al. (2013). Predicting date of birth and examining the best time to date a pregnancy. Int J Gynaecol Obstet, 123(2): 105–9.

123. Grobman, W. A., Rice, M. M., Reddy, U. M., et al. (2018). Labor induction versus expectant management in low-risk nulliparous women. N Engl J Med, 379: 513–523.

124. ACOG Practice Bulletin No. 146 (2014). Management of late-term and postterm pregnancies. Obstet Gynecol, 124(2 Pt 1): 390–6.

125. Rosenstein, M. G., Cheng, Y. W., Snowden, J. M., et al. (2012). Risk of stillbirth and infant death stratified by gestational age. Obstet Gynecol, 120(1): 76–82.

126. Stapleton, S. R., Osborne, C. and Illuzzi, J. (2013). Outcomes of care in birth centers: demonstration of a durable model. J Midwifery Womens Health, 58(1): 3–14.

Chapter Eight

127. Harari, Y. N. (2014). *Sapiens: A Brief History of Humankind*. Published in the U.K. by Harvill Secker First; published in Hebew in Israel in 2011 by Kinneret, Zmora-Bitan, Dvir.

128. Centers for Disease Control and Prevention (2018). Pregnancy Mortality Surveillance System. Division of Reproductive Health, National Center for Chronic Disease Prevention and Health Promotion. Available at: https://www.cdc.gov/reproductivehealth/maternalinfanthealth/pregnancy-mortality-surveillance-system.htm

129. Building U.S. Capacity to Review and Prevent Maternal Deaths (2018). Report from nine maternal mortality review committees. Available at: http://reviewtoaction.org/Report_from_Nine_MMRCs

130. Georgetown University. "How Does Race Impact Childbirth Outcomes?" FNP Program. Available at: https://online.nursing.georgetown.edu/blog/race-disparities-maternal-infant-outcomes/

131. Giscombé, C. L. and Lobel, M. (2005). Explaining disproportionately high rates of adverse birth outcomes among African Americans: The impact of stress, racism, and related factors in pregnancy. Psychol Bull, 131(5): 662–83.

132. Alhusen, J. L., Bower, K. M., Epstein, E., et al. (2016). Racial discrimination and adverse birth outcomes: An integrative review. J Midwifery Womens Health, 61(6): 707–720.

133. Harrell, J. P., Hall, S. and Taliaferro, J. (2003). Physiological responses to racism and discrimination: an assessment of the evidence. Am J Public Health, 93(2): 243–8.

134. Collins, J. W., Jr, David, R. J., Handler, A., et al. (2004). Very low birthweight in African American infants: the role of maternal exposure to interpersonal racial discrimination. Am J Public Health, 94(12): 2132–2138.

135. Yehuda, R. and Lehrner, A. (2018). Intergenerational transmission of trauma effects: putative role of epigenetic mechanisms. World Psychiatry, 17(3): 243–257.

136. David, R. J. and Collins, J. W. (1997). Differing birth

weight among infants of U.S.-born blacks, African-born blacks, and U.S.-born whites. N Engl J Med, 337(17): 1209–14.

137. Collins, J. W., Wu, S.-Y. and David, R. J. (2002). Differing intergenerational birth weights among the descendants of US-born and Foreign-born whites and African Americans in Illinois. Am J Epidemiol, 155(3): 210–6.

138. Brown, R. A., & Armelagos, G. J. (2001). Apportionment of racial diversity: A review. Evolutionary Anthropology, 10: 34–40.

139. Machery, E., & Faucher, L. (2005). Social construction and the concept of race. Phil Science, 72: 1208–1219.

140. Tatum, B. A. (2017). *Why are all the Black Kids Sitting Together in the Cafeteria?* Basic Books, Hachette Book Group: New York.

141. National Partnership for Women and Families. (2018). Issue Brief: Listening to Black Mothers in California. Available at: http://www.nationalpartnership.org/our-work/resources/health-care/maternity/listening-to-black-mothers-in-california.pdf

142. Vedam, S., Stoll, K., Taiwo, T. K. et al. (2019). The Giving Voice to Mothers Study: Inequity and mistreatment during pregnancy and childbirth in the United States. Reprod Health, 16(1):77.

143. Haskell, R. (2018). Serena Williams on Motherhood, Marriage, and Making Her Comeback. Vogue. Available at: https://www.vogue.com/article/serena-williams-vogue-cover-interview-february-2018

144. Nuru-Jeter, A., Dominguez, T. P., Hammond, W. P. et al. (2009). "It's the skin you're in": African-American women talk about their experiences of racism. Matern Child Health J 13(1): 29–39.

145. Wailoo, K. (2018). Historical aspects of race and medicine: The case of J. Marion Sims. JAMA, 320(15): 1529–1530.

146. Smith, S. G., Basile, K. C., Merrick, M. T., et al. (2018). The National Intimate Partner and Sexual Violence Survey (NISVS): 2015 Data Brief – Updated Release. Atlanta, GA: National Center for Injury Prevention and Control, Centers for Disease Control and Prevention. Available at: https://www.cdc.gov/violenceprevention/pdf/2015data-brief508.pdf

147. Ferguson v. Charleston, 532 U.S. 67 (2001). Available at https://supreme.justia.com/cases/federal/us/532/67/

Chapter Nine

148. Beck, C. T. and Gable, R. K. (2012). A Mixed Methods Study of Secondary Traumatic Stress in Labor and Delivery Nurses. J Obstet Gynecol Neonatal Nurs, 41(6): 747–60.

149. Pfifferling, J-H. and Gilley, K. (2000). Overcoming Compassion Fatigue. Fam Pract Manag, 7(4):39–44.

150. Greenfield, B. (2015). Bullied, powerless, and defeated: 45 women share their striking birth stories. Yahoo Parenting. Available at https://www.yahoo.com/news/bullied-powerless-and-defeated-45-women-share-123515276107.html

151. Siebert, V. (2015). Emotional photo essay reveals a darker side to the delivery room as mothers detail how they were 'bullied' by doctors during birth and 'forced' to undergo invasive procedures against their will. The Daily Mail. Available at https://www.dailymail.co.uk/femail/article-3155535/Emotional-photo-essay-reveals-darker-delivery-room-mothers-bullied-doctors-birth-forced-undergo-invasive-procedures-against-will.html

152. Covey, S., Merrill, A. R. and Merrill, R. R. (2015). *First Things First.* FranklinCovey Co. Mango Media Miami.

Chapter Ten

153. Weston, J. (2011). *Mastering Respectful Confrontation: A Guide to Personal Freedom and Empowered, Collaborative Engagement.* Heartwalker Press.

Chapter Eleven

154. Beck, C. T. and Watson, S. (2016). Posttraumatic growth after birth trauma: "I was broken, now I am unbreakable." MCN Am J Matern Child Nurs, 41(5): 264–71.

155. Norman Nathan, A. (2016). "Another nurse held my baby's head into my vagina to prevent him from being delivered." Cosmopolitan. Available at https://www.cosmopolitan.com/lifestyle/news/a62592/caroline-malatesta-brookwood-childbirth-lawsuit/

156. Tucker, S. Y. (2018). There is a hidden epidemic of doctors abusing women in labor, doulas say. Broadly (VICE). Available at https://www.vice.com/en_us/article/evqew7/obstetric-violence-doulas-abuse-giving-birth

157. Bregel, S. (2016). Alabama mom finally gets justice after traumatic birth left her permanently injured. Babble.com Available at https://www.babble.com/parenting/caroline-malatesta-alabama-mom-wins-law-suit-after-birth-injury/

158. For more information about the *Mother May I?* documentary film, visit https://mothermayithemovie.com

159. Pittman, T. (2018). Inside the documentary uncovering traumatic birth experiences. Huffington Post. Available at https://www.huffpost.com/entry/birth-trauma-mother-may-i-documentary_n_5b16adb5e4b0734a9937bf34

160. Pinker, S. and Morey. A. (2011). *The Better Angels of Our Nature: Why Violence Has Declined.* Viking Books.

Epilogue

161. McIntosh, P. (2003). White privilege: Unpacking the invisible knapsack. In S. Plous (Ed.), *Understanding prejudice and discrimination* (pp. 191–196). New York, NY, US: McGraw-Hill.

162. Irving, Debbie. (2014). *Waking up White, and Finding Myself in the Story of Race.* Elephant Room Press.

163. Tatum, B. A. (2017). *Why are all the Black Kids Sitting Together in the Cafeteria?* Basic Books, Hachette Book Group: New York.

164. Jacobs, H. A. (1861). *Incidents in the Life of a Slave Girl.*

165. Coates, T. N. (2015). *Between the World and Me.* Spiegel & Grau.

166. Pinker, S. and Morey. A. (2011). *The Better Angels of Our Nature: Why Violence Has Declined.* Viking Books.

167. Weston, J. (2011). *Mastering Respectful Confrontation: A Guide to Personal Freedom and Empowered, Collaborative Engagement.* Heartwalker Press.

About the Author

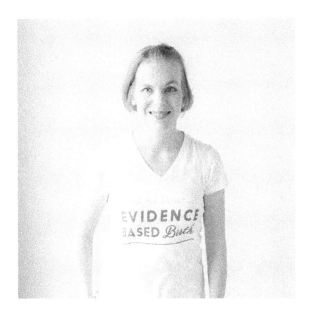

REBECCA DEKKER, PHD, RN, is the founder and CEO of Evidence Based Birth®. After earning her Bachelor's, Master's, and PhD in Nursing, Rebecca embarked on a career as a nurse scientist and teacher. In 2016, she left academia to become a full-time entrepreneur and consumer advocate for evidence based care. Rebecca lives in Lexington, Kentucky, where she and her husband Dan are raising three children and an assortment of pets. *Babies Are Not Pizzas* is her first book.

9 781732 549661